Notting Hill Editions is an independent British publisher. The company was founded by Tom Kremer (1930–2017), champion of innovation and the man responsible for popularising the Rubik's Cube.

After a successful business career in toy invention Tom decided, at the age of eighty, to fulfil his passion for literature. In a fast-moving digital world Tom's aim was to revive the art of the essay, and to create exceptionally beautiful books that would be lingered over and cherished.

Hailed as 'the shape of things to come', the family-run press brings to print the most surprising thinkers of past and present. In an era of information-overload, these collectible pocket-size books distil ideas that linger in the mind.

nottinghilleditions.com

Dr Andrew Lees is a Professor of Neurology at the National Hospital, Queen Square, London. He is the recipient of numerous awards, including the American Academy of Neurology Lifetime Achievement Award, the Gowers Medal, the Association of British Neurology and the British Neuropsychiatry Association medals and the Dingebauer Prize of the German Society of Neurology for outstanding research. He is one of the three most highly cited Parkinson's disease researchers in the world. He is the author of several books, including *Ray of Hope*, runner-up in the William Hill Sports Book of the Year; *The Silent Plague*; *Liverpool: The Hurricane Port*; the critically acclaimed *Mentored by a Madman: The William Burroughs Experiment* and, most recently, *Brazil That Never Was*, both published by Notting Hill Editions.

BRAINSPOTTING

Adventures in Neurology

–

A. J. Lees

 Notting Hill Editions

Published in 2022
by Notting Hill Editions Ltd
Mirefoot, Burneside, Kendal LA8 9AB

Series design by FLOK Design, Berlin, Germany
Cover design by Tom Etherington
Creative Advisor: Dennis PAPHITIS

Typeset by CB Editions, London
Printed and bound by Memminger MedienCentrum,
Memmingen, Germany

Cover illustration: Antony Gormley, BRAIN FIELD, 2007
Lithograph on 300 gsm Velin d'Arches paper, 100 x 69 cm
© the artist, courtesy White Cube

Image credits: p.19: *Clifford Wilson, Professor of Medicine, Lecturing at
The London Hospital, Whitechapel* by John Stanton Ward. © The Estate
of John Stanton Ward and Bridgeman Images. Courtesy of the Royal
London Hospital Archives; p.48: *A Clinical Lesson at the Salpêtrière*
(1887) by André Brouillet, reproduced by kind permission of Olivier
Walusinski and the Musée d'histoire de la medicine (University of Paris);
p.92: Maida Vale Hospital for Nervous Diseases. Courtesy of the Queen
Square Archives.

A CIP record for this book is available from the British Library.

ISBN 978-1-912559-36-7

nottinghilleditions.com

Contents

To my teachers

'My dear fellow,' said Sherlock Holmes as we sat on either side of the fire in his lodgings at Baker Street, 'life is infinitely stranger than anything which the mind of man could invent.'

– 'A Case of Identity' (1891), from *The Adventures of Sherlock Holmes* by Sir Arthur Conan Doyle

– Preface –

When I tell people I am a neurologist, very few have much idea of what I do. Common reactions are: 'Isn't that the same as Gregory House?' or 'How wonderful it must be to study the human mind?' When I reply that I make the blind see, the lame walk and can calm the shaking palsy, many assume I must be a brain surgeon. The media prefer to call me a 'leading neuroscientist' even though I spend no time in a laboratory and carry out no research on the healthy brain.

Neuroscience engages the attention and curiosity of the general public despite its complexity, and in the last twenty years various domains of knowledge have acquired a 'neuro' prefix that attempts to link them with the nervous system. Timothy Leary, the Harvard Professor of Psychology who advised my generation to 'turn on, tune in, drop out' with LSD-25, was the first person to link life science with culture, and there are now specialists in neuroaesthetics, neurotheology, neuroeconomics, neuromarketing and even neurolaw.

Neurology, the term coined by Thomas Willis in the seventeenth century to describe the doctrine of the nerves, now refers to the study and treatment of disorders of the nervous system. Although both neurology and psychiatry are concerned with disordered behaviour and thinking, a high wall has grown up between the two specialties that has proved very difficult to break down. Most psychiatrists insist that the patient's narrative matters in its own right without any requirement for spotlight consciousness. The neurological examination, on the other hand, reminds psychiatrists that in order to solve medical problems they need to observe as well as listen, and that a practical knowledge of the brain's morphology and physiology is important.

During my training, neurologists were held in awe for their clinical acumen and their uncanny ability to diagnose zebras and black swans, but equally they were caricatured by colleagues as introverted, analytical eggheads that combined the precision of mathematicians with the scrupulosity of bryologists and the sobriety of undertakers. Theirs was a young science in which expertise had been passed down often by word of mouth at the bedside, from master to master. These supermen, and they were all men, convinced me that it was only a matter of time before every brain disease would be categorised in terms of its anatomical, electrical and chemical connections, and that all mental life would be mapped to a neural substrate. Neurologists were literally the brains of the medical profession; their rational approach drew me in. My own first teachers emphasised that my training would be as long and demanding as that required of a vestal virgin in Ancient Rome: that I would need to listen, observe and infer and also learn the importance of contemplation. The method I used was reasoned and left little to the imagination.

It took ten years of apprenticeship before I felt competent to diagnose and treat most of the common neurological syndromes and even longer before I felt reasonably confident to distinguish a healthy person from an ill one. During my long career as a neurologist, I have treated about 30,000 patients in National Health Service clinics, and several thousand more in the consulting rooms at University College Hospital and the National Hospital, Queen Square, London. I have done about 4,000 ward rounds and seen hundreds of hospital referrals. I have taught undergraduate and postgraduate students at the bedside and in seminar rooms and have lectured to colleagues in large auditoria all over the world. I have visited patients in their own homes, although not as many as I would have liked. I have tried to find answers to the questions my patients asked me and which I was unable to answer at the time.

I mention these facts only to illustrate the difference between my medical life and the practice of Oliver Sacks, who, during his lifetime, became the best-known neurologist on the planet. In 1976 Jonathan Cole, a medical student at the Middlesex Hospital, wrote to Dr Sacks to see if he might spend a two-month elective in his department. After some delay and with some embarrassment Sacks wrote back apologetically saying that he no longer had a salaried post at Beth Abraham hospital, and that he was a neurological gypsy who survived marginally and precariously on odd jobs here and there. He was a physician without a post, a romantic scientist, more at home in the asylums of yesteryear than in the new skyscraper hospitals, but his letters – handwritten from his desk in Horatio Street, West Village, New York – gave renewed hope to the ignored, and his books made neurology more human. Through his writing Sacks was able to reconcile the afflicted with their environment. To many neurologists he came over more like a psychiatrist in the mould of Sigmund Freud.

I took a different course. I watched my ps and qs and hoped that I could contribute something worthwhile by working inside a healthcare system that I respected and looked up to. I avoided the cardinal sin of letting fantasy get the better of objectivity, and after twenty years I was rewarded with my own department. This allowed me to surround myself with brilliant colleagues and to be inspired by curious young minds. Their example sometimes allowed me to see bigger pictures and through their ideas acquire new ways of detecting disease.

I now work on a different scale and time course with redefined cultural constructions and contexts, but the medical interview and neurological examination have remained as vital as ever. The clinical method I describe throughout this book involves paying great attention to detail and has an applicability in reducing error that goes far beyond the diagnosis of disease, yet in spite of its great value it is no more than a type of accurate guessing in which the end point achieved is a name. Over time this name that is given to a collection of symptoms and signs comes to assume the importance of a specific entity, although it is never more than an insecure, ephemeral conception. After almost half a century of seeing people in the clinic, I still feel like an explorer shining a pocket torch into a cave and hoping I will find a precious stone. The careful study of a patient's symptoms from the beginning to the end of their disease remains my chosen animal model and I remain as committed to clinical trials, best evidence and the need for medical statistics as I was when I completed my training as a doctor. I am enamoured by the exciting new approaches to restoring function to the brain injured and by the way genetics has changed the face of neurology.

Despite continuous change in the classification of neurological disorders over the last four decades, the contents of my doctor's bag have hardly altered. I still carry an ophthalmoscope, a Queen Square hammer, a red hatpin, a 128 Hz tuning fork, a pin hole, a pen torch and some orange sticks. New additions are Neurotips for testing pain sensation, which have replaced pins, the 'little green book' for assessing cognition, and some applications on my mobile phone, such as the Ishihara test for colour vision, a Snellen's visual acuity chart and an electronic black-and-white-striped moving drum for testing optokinetic nystagmus.

Even after so long surprises occur in the clinic. Last year a married couple who are professional ballroom dancers came to see me. After immaculate synchronicity for twenty-five years, they had suddenly run into timing problems. The wife told me that her husband was now making one or two false steps, particularly when dancing the paso doble. As I then listened to his own account, which involved technical terms such as 'reduced horizontal energy', there was nothing that I could see that indicated a neurological problem. When it came to the examination I asked him to tap his feet on the ground one at a time and noticed that the movements of his right foot were more irregular, slower and less rhythmical than those on the left. I suspected Parkinson's disease but rather than ordering a dopamine transporter scan I told them that I was not sure what was wrong but that I wanted to see him again in three months' time. Hearing a new presentation of a common disease still gives me enormous pleasure and I added 'the faulty dance step' to my list of uncommon presentations of Parkinson's that already included 'swimming in circles', 'the Rolex watch that kept stopping', 'the white hand', the 'skiing smudge in the snow' and 'the foot cramp of the long-distance runner'.

My enthusiasm for eliciting physical signs is as strong as it ever was. I marvel at the pathognomonic, appreciate the cardinal, and adore even the softest of commemoratives. Some of the abnormalities I see and feel and then record indicate old scars; others are harbingers, but it is those that reveal the cause of the presenting complaint that I value most. I also like the menagerie similes including dromedary, hobby horse, dancing bear and cock to describe different pathological gaits, but these terms should not be used in front of patients.

When I started to write this book I was searching for a lost soulful neurology that arose out of the diverse and fascinating presentations of nervous disease and the richness of my speciality's accumulated literature. Through time-drifting and heart-searching I was able to randomly connect with the past and recall demonstrations from my apprenticeship that had helped to form my views about how neurology should be practised. I could also rely for source material on a handful of minor medical triumphs and a cemetery full of mistakes that had been etched deep in my memory. Insight allowed me to envisage a scintillating future that transcended representation and mechanisms, where the double helix and the enchanted loom merged with the magical universe to reveal the identity of illness.

– Birdwatching on the Pavements –

I still remember dreams where I could fly, and how as a child I loved the sound of a tawny owl hoot. Recognising a robin, a duck, a swan and a house sparrow was part of growing up, but I also picked up the names of other birds I didn't know from the chatter of my mother and father, as they looked over our little lawn at teatime. Every Thursday, when the box of groceries was delivered from the Thrift Store, I pulled out the packet of PG Tips and rummaged in its foil wrapper and cardboard carton hoping a Brooke Bond Tea collectable picture card of a gannet would fall out rather than yet another duplicate of a bird I already had. It was these cards that provided the platform for me to leave stamp collecting and trainspotting behind and start to create an inventory of living things.

For my twelfth birthday I asked for a compendium that would allow me to put a name to the birds I was seeing in my garden and the old pasture that sloped down from the bottom of our road. Every bird that had been sighted more than fifty times in the last hundred years was included in my *Collins Pocket Guide to British Birds*. Richard Fitter, its author, had discarded the standard Linnaean classification and devised a new approach that would assist birdwatchers out in the field to identify species they had only glimpsed. The manual's descriptive section was divided into the three broad habitats of land, waterside and water, and within each of these groupings the indigenous species were laid out in ascending order based on their length. The sixty-four pages of illustrations arranged the individual types by their colour and likeness while also depicting raptors, gulls and waders in flight. At the bottom of each plate there was a silhouette of a house sparrow, which served as a size comparator, and in the key at the back birds were categorised according to the colour of their feathers, anatomical features such as their feet, head, wings and tail, their haunts, and particular behavioural characteristics. The guide made the point that female, male and immature birds of the same variety could look quite different and that plumage often changed markedly with the season. It also reassured me that even expert birdwatchers, in their mania for rarities, made diagnostic errors.

One day, about a year after I had started to keep records, I looked out from my bedroom window on to the rugby pitch and saw a group of dark birds huddled close to the twenty-five-yard line. In a moment of drama, they rocketed into the air, skimming the tops of the goalposts, and whirred away over the chimney tops. The pack of eight were back the following morning, crouched low on the grass pecking the pitch like pigeons with their small black beaks. My mother and father could neither tell me their name, nor where they had come from.

There were too many medium-sized land birds in my guide to be of much help and none of the illustrations seemed to be a close match for what I was seeing. So, I turned to the key. The list of brown birds included partridge, woodcock, corncrake, snipe, ruff and bittern, but only two of them, the golden plover and the red grouse, had a black bill. I flipped back through the illustrations and immediately discounted the plover, so I homed in on the red grouse. The text informed me that *Lagopus lagopus scotica* was endemic to the upland moors of the British Isles where it fed on ling, bilberries and small insects. Field identifiers that I had been unable to discern included a crimson band above the eye, a hook-tipped bill and light-grey feathered feet. Sensing my uncertainty, my father reminded me that birds could fly anywhere they wanted to and that very few remained in one place for long. He went on to say, with a smile on his face, 'Birds also do not read bird books.' That evening I wrote in my diary:

The red grouse were on the rugby pitch. I think they may have come here to escape the burning heather on Blubberhouses Moor.

The identification of the red grouse sparked my interest and I started to spend Saturdays travelling to bird haunts like Spurn Head and Swillington Ings in the company of adult naturalists. These experienced and generous people emphasised to me the importance of writing down what I saw and showed me where and how to look.

My mother, who sometimes used birds to tell fortunes, conserved my bird journals for many years. After I had qualified as a doctor she handed them back to me, reminding me how as a twelve-year-old I had felt the need to be able to name every little brown bird that came into view. She then said, 'Do you remember when you found that dead blue tit unmarked in the garden and how you buried it under the laburnum, marking its resting place with an ice lolly stick?' At the time she had told me that when sailors were lost at sea blue tits carried their souls to heaven.

I have one of my old maroon hardback journals open in front of me now, its lined pages filled with an italic script that I scarcely recognise as my own. Each entry is meagre and ordinary; the mechanical accounting with daily averages and graphs that followed the descriptions were remnants of my need for systems, formality and rules. Even so, watching birds had taught me the virtue of patience and composure and how to focus on a single living thing at the expense of everything around it:

Sunday April 24th
The weather was cold with a strong wind blowing . . . A blue tit was feeding on the nuts when a greenfinch wanted to. A

fight broke out but not for long for the tit attacked the finch with such ferocity that the greenfinch was forced to withdraw.

Saturday June 11th
The weather was mild but there were a few rain showers. A song thrush began to build a nest in the flowering currant bush, but it was only seen once. It probably still had some young to feed and was building the new nest in its spare time.

Daltonism, caused by a mutation in the green pigment in the cones of my retina, was an inconvenience that forced me to rely more heavily on the size, shape and behaviour of a bird than the colour of its feathers. My parents had told me that the grouse on the rugby pitch were chestnut, rather than just dark, giving me the missing marker that had allowed me to identify them in my vade mecum. Flashes of buffs and greens that were so important in distinguishing dun female dabbling ducks like mallards, gadwalls, pintails and teals were beyond my visual range and I was forced to focus on movement and learn to spot an immature blackbird just by the way she cocked her head. When a dark shape dropped like a stone from the garden fence, I did not need to see a red breast to know it had to be a robin. I became an expert in the 'jizz' of birds and was soon able to put a name to many of them just from their flight or the way they walked or hopped. I also discovered through my interactions with other bird watchers that I was better than everyone else at picking up birds hidden in long grass. When out of the corner of my eye I spotted a mouse-rustle in fallen leaves I knew that if it was tiny, chunky and brown with a cocked tail it was a wren, while if it was the size of a house sparrow with a streaked back and moved with a nervy shuffle, flicking its wings, it just had to be a dunnock. One of the naturalists who had taught me how to tell a willow warbler from a chiffchaff, and was aware of my colour blindness, told me that in World War II colour-deficient observers had been able to penetrate the khaki camouflage of the enemy when it had deceived able-sighted people.

At fifteen my father introduced me to the *Selected Poems* of John Clare. In the introduction, Geoffrey Grigson wrote that as a young man Clare had scraped a living as a farm labourer in the fields, worked as a potboy at the Blue Bell public house and then as a gardener on the Burghley Estate. He learned to play the fiddle with gypsies near his home in the village of Helpston and later enrolled in the militia, but by the age of fourteen he had fallen in love with the written word. When he could not afford writing material he used birch bark as papyrus and a mix of bruised nut galls, green copper and bluestone soaked in a pint and a half of rainwater for ink.

As he wandered in the flatlands between limestone outcrop and Fen and the wooded hillsides around Helpston, the remedial currents of nature helped to calm his dread of enclosure and confirmed his identity. He wrote to feel happier and to calm an impending sense of loss. Each of his poems was a point of departure. In order to get closer to birds and go deeper into their lives he would hide in the long, wet grass, scramble on all fours under bushes, wade through swamps and scale ancient oaks. He watched wisps of snipe standing in clumps of yellow flags in wetland, nightjars whirling over the furze and a pair of ravens nesting in a giant oak. He wrote that the world's end was at the edge of the horizon and that a day's journey was enough to carry him to its brink from where he could look down and see heaven in the sea. He stalked a circle, losing himself in the misty blue, but he always returned home. The informality of his verse made it seem as if he was sharing his deepest secrets with me.

Clare's poems gave intimate information about the locations of birds' nests and the grasses, moss, twigs, hairs and mud used to construct them. The fragility and decorativeness of eggs fascinated him, the yellowhammer's 'scribbled as with ink and pen' and the 'deadened green' of the nightingale's clutch that he had found concealed in a bush of thorns. As he idled on common ground, melodious lyrics flowed in his head:

> The crowds of starnels whizz and hurry by,
> And darken like a clod the evening sky:
> The larks like thunder rise and suther round
> Then drop and nestle in the stubble ground . . .

His knowledge of bird call meant that he was able to appreciate the drama going on in the trees and his sensitive ear allowed him to transcribe, rather than translate, the nightingale's song:

—'Chew-chew chew-chew' & higher still
'Cheer-cheer, cheer-cheer' more loud and shrill . . .
'Wew-wew wew-wew chur-chur chur-chur
Woo-it woo-it'—could this be her
'Tee-rew tee-rew tee-rew tee-rew
Chew-rit chew-rit'—& ever new
'Will-will will-will grig-grig grig-grig'

Clare knew nature by heart. Birds recognised him, and he belonged with them. Those he encountered on his rambles became part of his very being. Sometimes he used graphic local names like butter bump for bittern, fire tail for redstart, fern owl for nightjar and bumbarrel for the long-tailed tit, and his eye for detail drew my attention to things I had never noticed. He likened the cuckoo to a hawk in flight, commented on its red mouth and sharp eye and how in June it forgot its song; his pureness of vision seemed to make the birds I had watched even more alive. In spite of his deep knowledge of the natural world he always rejected the 'dark system' of Latinate names that he believed stripped birds from their culture:

I love to see the nightingale in its hazel retreat and the Cuckoo hiding in its solitudes of oaken foliage and not to examine their carcasses in glass cases, yet naturalists & botanists seem to have no taste for this poetical feeling they merely make collection of dried specimens classing them after Linnaeus into tribes and families.

Nature's stability was now providing me with a refuge. After the rains of May and the sunshine of June I turned my attention to the life that depended for its survival on the desolate pasture. As I lay in the long grass listening to the rasp and scrape of grasshoppers, a skylark darted out of the sward and climbed into the air. Each ascent that I observed in the coming days was like a firework display engineered to stunning effect, but one which varied in its calculated spontaneity and depended on the weather. The more I observed birds the more I became aware of their allure and the beauty contained within their ordinariness. Bird watching had become a vigil comparable to prayer and Clare had added poetry to my science:

Let the naturalist catch the glow-worm, carry it home with him in a box, and find it next morning nothing but a little grey worm; let the poet visit it at evening, when beneath the scented hawthorn and the crescent moon it has built itself a palace of emerald light.

What surprises me most as I read my childhood journals is that they are devoid of not just colour but also song. It was as if I had been deaf to the calls of birds and that I had needed to see their fluttering shapes to be certain they existed. Yet as I cast my mind back to those halcyon days, it is the harmonious discord of birds that evokes my sweetest memories of our garden and the dark wood, the four-note lullaby of the wood pigeon, the death rattle of magpies and the cuckoo I never saw. A year after I had found John Clare the diggers and steamrollers came over the tops, and a gleaming new housing estate with high-rise blocks and semi-detached palaces stood where the skylarks had once plummeted to earth: the meadow was now a transformed landscape of lost freedom.

My field journals had got me started with cataloguing and organising knowledge, and through mixing with learned men at a young age I came to realise that a familiarity of observation was the essence of all natural history. Furthermore, my colour blindness had taught me that a perceived deficit could sometimes be associated with compensatory biological advantage, including a greater appreciation of texture and contrast. And then Clare had introduced me to the incredible power of passive attentiveness and showed me a new way to make birds visible on the written page.

At the age of twenty-two I was interested first and foremost in the accurate diagnosis of each medical species, the habitats and behaviour of patients and the study of remedies derived from plants. I had started to enjoy the nineteenth-century descriptions of illness by novelists such as Zola and Flaubert as well as the medical accounts of disease by physicians like William Heberden, James Paget and Richard Bright. It was the natural history of medicine, rather than a desire to save lives, or even search for disease causation, that kept me motivated.

During my training, the intellectual challenge of neurology and the inherent logic of its method appealed to me. I liked the idea that by listening attentively to the distress calls of patients I could determine the source of their complaint, and that by thoroughly examining them I could localise the site of their lesion. As more data filtered in from tests I was then able to infer the likely cause by a stepwise process of elimination. Instead of looking at size and shape, colour and distinctive field marks as I did when birding, I inspected each patient for stiffness and weakness and the presence of any adventitious involuntary movements. The pill-rolling rest tremor of Parkinson's disease was akin to the kestrel's hover. I recalled how I had often tried to photograph an unusual bird that had refused to stay still and had not been able to capture enough key features to identify it with certainty, and I noticed how similar the process was to listening to a collection of baffling symptoms when the features of the underlying disease had not yet declared themselves.

Once I had become a junior doctor competent and knowledgeable enough to educate medical students, I tried to involve them rather than force them to listen, but when teaching at the bedside I would pin them down to say categorically whether what they had observed was pathological or within the normal range, and whether the totality of their findings could be explained by a single focus of damage. When we were short of instructive cases on the ward I took them round the Circle Line. Before leaving the Cruciform Building on Gower Street I asked them to observe the Underground passengers surreptitiously, paying particular attention to facial expression and hands and feet, observing how they rose on leaving the carriage and how they walked down the platform. I stressed to them that they needed to melt into the background and try to become invisible. After buying the tickets at the Euston Square ticket office we went downstairs to the westbound platform and when the next train pulled in, we split up and entered four different compartments. It took just over an hour to go full circle. On returning to the day room, I asked them to give me a statement of what they had seen, much as they might do to the London Transport police after witnessing a crime. I expected them to comment on the subject's likely ethnic origin and, if they had heard any speech, the likely place of upbringing. If the person who had become the focus of their gaze had bright or beady eyes I asked if they had been able to note the size of the pupil. If the passenger had looked anxious or angry I asked them to try to explain what it was that had made them think that. If they had noticed a person with a limp on leaving the carriage I pushed them for more descriptive detail. I was pleased when they embellished their account with observations relating to the individual's clothes and accoutrements or when they speculated about the individual's likely occupation. My intention was to try to encourage them to become doctors on whom nothing would be lost.

Although we never discussed possible medical diagnoses, I also wanted them to become aware that a clinical picture was far more than just a sick person in a nightdress lying in a hospital bed. The red grouse had taught me that when common things have been eliminated I should never be afraid to diagnose the exotic or unexpected; binoculars had taught me the power of instrumentation and I was never without my ophthalmoscope in clinic. Retracting an incorrect diagnosis had far more serious repercussions than a bird spotting error and despite the appeal of pattern recognition I refrained from instant diagnosis and always acted as my own devil's advocate. Bird watching had also alerted me to the challenging problem posed by mimics and by phenotypic variation. For example Huntington's disease, that usually presented in later life with chorea, depression and cognitive impairment, could present in the young with a slowness and stiffness that resembled Parkinson's disease, and migraine chameleons included stroke, epilepsy and vestibular disorders.

At medical school in the late nineteen-sixties my nature walks became dérives. Even now as I walk I am always trying to better understand the habitats and lives of the people I encounter in the sanctuary of the hospital. If I meet my patients in the street I want to be able to not just recognise them, but to be able to talk to them about things other than their health. It took a long time for me to appreciate that giving a name to a disease was in fact the easiest part of good neurological practice. In order to make people better, neurologists need to bring themselves – as well as their tool kit – to the consultation. I still keep my eyes open for a black redstart on the Soho rooftops and for patients with chronic and debilitating neurological illnesses I occasionally recommend 'bird therapy'.

– Full of East End Promise –

Written on the tombstone next to my grandpa's grave were the words: IN SOME NEW BRAIN THE SLEEPING DUST WILL WAKEN, an epitaph that encouraged me to go on believing that death was a prolonged slumber. Before I went to The London Hospital Medical College in Whitechapel I had never seen a corpse. Death was hidden in our family and was something that happened to birds and old people.

Six to a cadaver we stood motionless in gleaming white coats clutching our dissecting manuals. Mr Wolynski, aged sixty-seven, looked as if he had been in a fight. His eyes were wide open and his hair was stuck to his scalp with what looked like coagulated blood. When I touched his arms they felt like sculpted damp clay. Lashman, my dissecting partner, mumbled: 'This is how we will all end up.' As I began to clean and trace in the axilla reflecting fascia with my scalpel, one of the surgical demonstrators told me to try to visualise the relationships of the exposed tissues and remember their relative depths from the skin surface.

Each afternoon in my first pre-clinical year I scurried back to the West End to devote my evenings to the study of the anatomy of the human body. My cell had a single bed, a washbasin, a wardrobe with a glass mirror and an electric fire fastened to the wall. After washing my hands to try to remove the musty sickliness of Wolynski's embalmed body I began my nightly task of learning by rote the shape, the origins and insertions, the nerve supply and the function of each pair of skeletal muscles. I then tried to picture in my mind their surface anatomy with the aid of a poster of Charles Atlas, the Italian-American bodybuilder. New words like distal and proximal, anterior and posterior, ventral and dorsal, medial and lateral, rostral and caudal, superior and inferior were included in the obligatory burden of text used by anatomists to describe the topography of arteries and veins which I had exposed in Mr Wolynski's bloodless flesh. Lewd mnemonics like 'As She Lay Flat Oscar's Penis Slowly Mounted' helped me to memorise the branches of his external carotid artery and 'Two Zombies Buggered My Cat' the divisions of his facial nerve. Cryptic formulas like $LR_6(SO_4)_3$ (Lateral Rectus supplied by the 6th cranial nerve), SO (Superior Oblique supplied by the 4th cranial nerve), and the remaining extraocular muscles all supplied by the 3rd cranial nerve, and acronyms such as DAB (dorsal abductors) and PAD (palmar adductors) were used to remember the function of the different interossei muscles in his hand.

By the beginning of the second term, in January, the twelve dead people who slept in the anatomy department had departed and all I saw when I entered the dissection room were stale formaldehyde stiffs with vandalised limbs and eviscerated torsos. The mask, which guards the intimate parts of the human body, had been peeled away, forcing me to confront my own eventual decomposition. Dismemberment was a hallowed initiation rite for the study of medicine, which had changed little since the days of Leonardo and Vesalius. The location of The London Hospital in the poorest part of the capital meant that there had always been a plentiful supply of unclaimed paupers and foreign seamen for its surgeons to cut up. The L-plan college museum in the medical school was filled with surgical specimens in pots and jars and on its lower level the skeleton of Joseph Merrick (the Elephant Man) housed in a glass case cast his atmospheric presence over our seminars.

In the knitwork of terraced streets behind the hospital I often saw people with physical handicaps and disfigurements. There was a small woman in a shawl with no nose, a tramp with a lump the size of an orange on the top of his head and an elderly man with a bamboo spine that pivoted him forwards in a way that made it appear as if his head was being controlled by a marionette string. One day on Stepney Way I was surprised to see a man with trousers far too short for him walking backwards towards me as he smoked a cigarette.

In contrast to the medical college where I spent the first two years of my apprenticeship, the hospital was a hurly-burly place where groups of people bustled, paused and intermingled, regrouped and moved on. Nurses with status defined by the colour of their uniforms, midwives in blue, lithe physiotherapists, laboratory technicians carrying wire baskets full of rubber-bunged test tubes, smartly dressed porters pushing patients in wheelchairs, doctors in white coats in earnest conversation, patients on crutches, patients on stretchers and anxious families clutching bunches of flowers crowded the main corridor.

My clinical tutors reminded me that medicine was a calling requiring self-sacrifice and courage. A physician's work was to prevent disease, relieve suffering and, if possible, cure the sick. Treatment should be evidential, but clinical care was always personal and intimate. They stressed to me that when there was no cure a good character and kindness were powerful healing forces. Sir Robert Hutchison's famous petition to God was our devotion:

From inability to let well alone, from too much zeal for the new and contempt for what is old, from putting knowledge before wisdom, science before art and cleverness before common sense, from treating patients as cases and from making the cure of the disease more grievous than the endurance of the same, good Lord deliver us.

Wolynski had been my first patient and his death had provided me with restitution and a lasting feeling

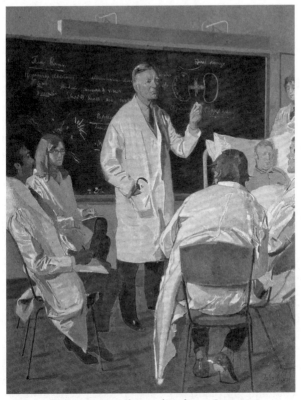

Clifford Wilson, Professor of Medicine, Lecturing at
The London Hospital, Whitechapel by John Stanton Ward.

of gratitude. The intricacy of his brachial plexus
reminded me of the exquisite workmanship of life
and, in the course of compiling a carnal index of his
vital structures, I had felt both respect and a sense of
obligation. I imagined him looking out to sea from the
deck of a freighter dreaming of what would never be,

but I also had nightmares that he had been cornered in an alleyway in Wapping by a group of snarling men with bottles.

Although medical students were not directly involved in clinical care I was encouraged to discuss my findings with the house officer and my case notes were inserted into the dossier. In comparison with the official records my version of the patient's story was copious, less structured and replete with what were considered irrelevancies. Once or twice, though, I noticed glaringly obvious things that the junior doctors looking after the patient had overlooked.

The twelve-bedded Nightingale Wards of The London Hospital were full of patients with physical signs of serious illness. George Kensit, a fifty-five-year-old man, let out a crackling rattling noise each time he breathed that could be heard at the end of the ward. Shortness of breath had forced him to retire from his job making fireproof mattresses in Barking and he had been admitted to the hospital because he had started coughing up blood. As I got up to leave, he thanked me, and asked me to apologise to the Doc 'for being a trouble'. After I had presented his case my tutor puffed hard on his pipe and told me that the Cape Asbestos Factory where Kensit had worked was an industrial killing machine. For years the company had told their workers that provided they drank half a pint of milk a day they would be protected from the dust. Unlike most of the diseases I would encounter in the next three years asbestosis was man-made and preventable.

On my second medical firm the senior registrar decided to teach us about diabetes mellitus. He began by saying that the word 'diabetes' was Greek for 'siphon' but that the Romans had added the Latin word 'mellitus' for 'sweet' because they had observed that bees were strongly attracted to the urine of its thirsty victims. He then went into the sluice room, came out with a sample, and proceeded to dip his finger into the yellow-coloured excretion before sucking it and suggesting, by his facial expression, that it tasted sweet. He then asked us all to do the same. After we had tasted the urine he looked at us triumphantly and said: 'Today you have learned an important clinical lesson. None of you noticed that I dipped my middle finger into the urine but licked my index finger.' During my training, anecdotes were not scorned as some sort of inferior, unreliable evidence but were valued as an efficient way of grasping new knowledge. We were told that personal testimony had been the first step in many important medical discoveries and that it could carry significance far beyond the particulars it recounted.

Whitechapel Road was a grand boulevard, which served as the vena cava for the circulation coming into the heart of the city from Essex. The underground station on its north side resembled an old-fashioned picture house nestled between family-owned shops such as Wally for Wireless and King's Watchmaker and Jeweller. Above the portal into the Tube was a solicitor's office where I often watched secretaries typing away at their desks. The Waste, opposite the hospital, was alive with Cockney backchat and the cries of costermongers. Paul, who owned the record stall where I bought my first Marvin Gaye album, had a smoke hanging from his lower lip and a dustbin filled with blazing wood to keep him warm. A record was always playing on his small turntable as I browsed through his wooden boxes. On the rare occasions he spoke to me it seemed as if his voice was coming out of someone else's mouth.

Whitechapel in the late sixties was still an enclave with a very distinctive atmosphere informed by the substantial Jewish community which lived there. Often the high street was populated by men with side-curls, dressed in wide-brimmed black homburgs, below-the-knee black coats and shining white shirts; others were dressed in trilby hats and well-cut shabby suits carrying briefcases under their arms and speaking Yiddish to one another as they walked purposefully in the direction of Bethnal Green. Bangladeshis and Bengalis had just started to move into Brick Lane and an old French Huguenot church had been converted into a mosque, while the first halal butcher had arrived to compete with the kosher meat trade. On a visit to one of the first Indian restaurants called The Punjab, which had recently opened close to the hospital, I noticed that my waiter's hands and teeth were stained reddish black, which I learned was caused by chewing the betel nut, an Asian symbol of love that reputedly had a kick six times that of a double espresso but was as carcinogenic as the Cape Asbestos Factory in Barking.

At the end of my first clinical year the time came to present a case at the Friday circus nicknamed 'Henson's Half Hour' (ironically named after the title of the comedian Tony Hancock's television programme). Dr Ronald Henson was Lord Brain's protégé, a man reputed to have been of few words but with a capacious intellect, and the medical students saw his teaching sessions as a daunting but exciting challenge. I began my presentation in the manner I had been taught:

Mr Sammy Boyd is a sixty-two-year-old jeweller who has a shop on Whitechapel Road. Three months ago he began to slur his words and found it harder to swallow. He also started to weep uncharacteristically when watching Hollywood films. Shortly before his admission a concerned client had asked him whether he was drunk. Mr Boyd is receiving treatment for high blood pressure from his general practitioner and has chronic bronchitis. He lives in a small, terraced house in Bethnal Green, smokes ten cigarettes a day, rarely drinks alcohol and has two grown-up children.

Dr Henson had told us on a previous occasion that he could tell exactly what level of training each of us had reached by the precision of our clinical presentation, and as I spoke I was acutely aware of him summing me up. After I finished speaking he said very little and proceeded to the examination. When he had descended down the nervous system as far as the lower cranial nerves he beckoned his class to come forward so they could see for themselves that Mr Boyd's tongue was alive below its surface with what resembled a nest of rippling pinworms. This physical sign is called fibrillation and indicates damage to the nerve supply to the tongue muscle. His tongue was also thin and wasted, his gag reflex absent and his jaw jerk pathologically brisk. Dr Henson then asked Mr Boyd to carry out a few spoken and written commands and to name some common objects. When asked to repeat the tongue twisters 'Methodist Episcopal Church', 'British Constitution' and 'Baby Hippopotamus', it was evident to us that his speech was slow and indistinct. Dr Henson then asked me whether I thought his difficulty speaking was due to a disorder of language, articulation or phonation to which I replied that I thought it likely to be a problem with enunciation rather than with word finding. After Mr Boyd had been thanked for coming down and taken back to Paulin Ward we discussed the findings. Dr Henson concluded that it was almost certain that Mr Boyd had motor neurone disease but there was still a slender hope that the investigations would turn up a rare treatable mimic. He ended by telling us that motor neurone disease meant helplessness, despair and ultimate death, a diagnosis that should never be given unless there was absolute certainty. The theatricality of the occasion combined with Dr Henson's logical and ruthlessly rational approach appealed to me.

I also enjoyed psychiatry and particularly the instruction of Dr John Denham at Mile End Hospital. Denham told us that he had been taught before the war by a Viennese psychiatrist called Julius Wagner-Jauregg, who had won the Nobel Prize for curing neurosyphilis with malaria in a treatment that became known as pyrotherapy. He joked that it was the only example in medical history where one fatal illness had been used to treat another one. Denham had read all of Freud's works and emphasised that the content of mental suffering mattered and that the patient should always be centre stage. During one teaching round I remember he drew our attention to the characteristic behaviours, attitudes and postures assumed by people in long-stay institutions. To illustrate what he was trying to describe he got up and walked forwards robotically with drooping shoulders, neck flexed and with his hands held meekly in front of his body. He believed this hangdog appearance to be caused by extreme passivity resulting from isolation and loss of identity. On another occasion he told us that Collis Browne's chlorodyne used both as a cough medicine and to relieve diarrhoea contained liberal amounts of laudanum and chloroform and at just twenty-seven pence a bottle was now being bought at chemists on the Whitechapel Road by the growing number of East End heroin addicts as a top-up for their habit. He also spoke to us enthusiastically about the new major tranquilisers like Largactil that he believed would allow some schizophrenics to leave mental hospitals and live independently.

As I rotated through the different hospital departments, I came to realise that although medicine aspired to be a science, it was full of hasty generalisations and imperfect observations. Some of the diva doctors gave their opinion to the patients as if it were a divine gift while others, incapable of admitting failure, hid their inadequacy by the use of Greek and Latin euphemisms. I disliked their effete snobbery and hubris which sometimes caused dreadful disasters to happen and their use of words to describe medical conditions like 'idiopathic' and 'essential' that were meaningless ploys used to conceal ignorance. But there were other consultants who I warmed to: mentors who emphasised how important it was that a doctor should question every action and that rules must be broken if, in all good conscience, it was felt that by doing so a life could be saved. These happy givers helped me to make sense of things that seemed unjust and unfair and taught me that it was better to believe in remedial nonsense than adhere to therapeutic nihilism. They loved their work and made me understand that there was no place in medicine for a pessimist. A doctor must care for altruistic reasons, maintain equanimity, be generous, tolerant and decisive, and also keep a sense of humour. They also warned me that although it would be necessary to acquire a lot of facts there was a danger of being over-educated and under-cultivated.

Sid's was a few doors down from The Grave Maurice public house on the Whitechapel Road and a popular barber for modernists. On my first visit I asked him for a blow wave, only to be told my hair was too thin and soft. After trying unsuccessfully to create a centre parting with lacquer and a smattering of Brylcreem he tried to console me by saying, 'The good thing is you'll never go bald.' When we got to know each other better he started to tell me snippets of his life. His sister, Miriam, had been on a milk diet for a year waiting for Mr Hermon-Taylor to carry out a vagotomy and pyloroplasty and was in dreadful pain. I recommended liquorice and ginger. Every Tuesday evening he and a group of Bethnal Green cronies took the bus up to the dog track at Walthamstow to have a few bets and a drink. I still remember that Estelle's Folly and Bill the Pig, both trained by Tom Reilly, were his two favourite greyhounds. One of the jokes he told me was about a doctor doing his rounds on the lung cancer ward. After the doctor had informed the first patient, a Roman Catholic, that there was nothing else he could do to help him, the patient asked if he could see a priest to make a confession. The second patient, a Protestant, was also terminal and when the doctor asked him for his last wish he requested to see his family in order to say goodbye. The third was an elderly Jewish man with dropsy. 'And what is your last wish?' the doctor enquired. The old man turned to him and whispered, 'I'd like to see another doctor.' My appointments always ended with Sid removing the cape, showing me the back of my head with his mirror, brushing me down and helping me put my jacket back on before muttering conspiratorially: 'Anything for the weekend, sir?'

Down the road from Sid's, inside the dark interior of The Blind Beggar, there was a jukebox that always reminded me of the bonnet of a Cadillac, with its curved windscreen, tail fins and sunburst chromium grin. On Saturday lunchtimes from my seat by the window I would watch pods of back-combed pilots in fishtail parkas scooting to the west, all gleaming chrome and whipping aerial, with their girls pushing backwards on the pillions. The rich tapestry of Whitechapel added vividness to my medical studies in much the same way John Clare's poems had reinvigorated my birding.

Medicine was not simply a college course and what happened outside the hospital had the potential to affect what occurred within it. But also, I was genuinely curious about my patient's lives. If something affected them then it ought to affect me too. I wanted to try to put myself in their shoes and I knew that I needed to be out on the streets observing and listening as well as clerking patients on the wards. I started to pick up Yiddish by listening to the customers at Grodzinski's Bakery on Fieldgate Street and Sid later explained the difference between a *schnorrer*, a *schlepper*, a *schlemiel* and a *mashugana*, and the translation of *tochas* and *drek*. I also picked up Cockney rhyming slang like 'Danny' (Danny Marr) for 'car', 'Cut and Carried' for 'married' and 'Godfer' (God forbid) for 'kid' from the black cabbies at the pie and mash shop on Cambridge Heath Road. I inhaled Whitechapel's foreign smells of salt beef, sauerkraut, smoked turkey, herring and pastrami and revelled in the Spitalfields Market patter aimed at 'the ones born every day'. Whitechapel was full of sharp-witted individualists and the perfect milieu to study medicine.

– Charcot's Parrot –

I n the course of my rotation through the different specialties at The London Hospital I had learnt about Charcot's joint, his biliary triad, his crystals seen under the microscope in asthma and finally his eponymous neurological diseases. In the second half of the nineteenth century, Jean-Martin Charcot's second sight had allowed him to see patterns of disease that no one before him had ever noticed and after I had finished my house jobs and become a doctor I left London with the intention of walking him back to life. I arrived in Paris in 1972 to continue my medical training and hoping that I could learn to perceive things my mind did not yet know.

I set off early beneath a sky rendered oppressive by the first suns of June. A south-westerly wind had swept away the clouds and above the city mist hung an azure wall. At the Pont de la Tournelle I stopped for a moment to watch the yawning river as it flowed on its journey to the blue roofs of Rouen. The cast iron gate of Le Jardin des Plantes was closed, but through its filigree I could see the allées where the naturalist Georges Cuvier had imagined a dinosaur from a single bone. I left the embankment at the Austerlitz termi-

nus and sidled up the long boulevard that followed the
Métro in the direction of the Hôpital de la Salpêtrière.

Charcot had first appreciated the opportunities for
research at L'Hospice de la Vieillesse-Femmes de
la Salpêtrière during the final year of his internship.
In his thesis, in which he described how to distinguish chronic rheumatism from gout, he outlined the
anatomo-clinical method that would be fundamental
to all his future work. Practising nosography, as he
referred to it, depended on the meticulous correlation
of symptoms and signs with pathology. The first step
was to document in detail the history and clinical signs
over the extent of a person's illness and then examine
the brain and spinal cord after death. On leaving La
Salpêtrière to continue his medical training, Charcot
is reputed to have said: 'I must return here one day
and then stay.'

His next post was back at Hôpital de la Charité
where he had worked as Pierre Rayer's intern in 1851.
Rayer was an outstanding diagnostician and anato-
mist with a particular interest in kidney disease who
had recently been appointed Dean of the Faculty of
Medicine in Paris. He had a strong interest in pathology and had also been elected as the first President of
the Société de biologie. Impressed by his ability, Rayer
proposed Charcot as a titular member of the society
which provided his young assistant with the opportunity to present his scientific research in front of the

greatest naturalists and physiologists of Paris. During this second spell at Hôpital de la Charité Charcot was promoted to associate professor, and at the age of thirty-seven, with the support of Rayer, he finally achieved the promotion he had been hoping for and was appointed *chef de service* at La Salpêtrière.

The hospice owed its name to its origin as a magazine for saltpetre. After several gunpowder explosions the arsenal was relocated, and its former site converted into a poorhouse for women. By the time of the First French Republic (1792–1804), it had expanded into a vast repository for every sort of female social misfit. The insane were shackled in rat-infested dungeons and fed through iron grilles. There was a block where orphans and the children of the destitute lived until they were old enough to go out to work in factories and some of its inmates had been admitted against their will on the whim of their husbands. It was a threatening world of its own, described in the newspapers as 'The Versailles of Pain'.

By the time Jean-Martin Charcot returned to take charge in 1862, the criminals and most of the beggars had been moved to other facilities. It was still a dreaded, alien place, but little by little it had been transformed from the pandemonium of bedlam to a self-supporting colony. The residents of the hospice could be divided into three broad groups: elderly, frail women from the least favoured classes of society, whom desertion or ill fortune had placed under the protection of public charity; women of all ages with infirmity due to chronic incurable physical maladies; and lastly the mentally disturbed or inadequate. Shortly after he had returned to the hospice Charcot famously wrote about its research opportunities:

The clinical types available for study are represented by numerous examples, which enable us to study categorical disease during its entire course, so to speak, since the vacancies that occur in any specific disease are quickly filled in the course of time. We are, in other words, in possession of a sort of museum of living pathology of which resources are great.

With the assistance of his close friend and colleague Alfred Vulpian, he began at once to delineate the illnesses of all 2,635 female residents that were under their joint care, a project he would continue until his death thirty years later. Each morning he arrived promptly at the hospice in his carriage and drove through the Mazarin gate. After alighting and giving his two horses some sugar he walked across the courtyard to his office on the ground floor of the old Pariset division. It was here, on weekdays, that he would see patients brought to him from the wards, and each Sunday at 9.30 a.m. he taught his assistants using cases they had selected from the previous week's admissions from the clinic. The spartan room had dark walls, a single window, a few chairs, a small table and a wardrobe. Rubens and Raphael reproductions hung on the wall. The first teaching case would be brought in and his nurse would proceed to remove the patient's gown and nightdress. The intern then presented *l'observation* while Charcot sat drumming his fingers impatiently on the table. After a loaded pause, he might ask the patient a question about her family history or command her to make a movement. His penetrating gaze remained fixed on the scene in front of him. Then, following what seemed like an interminable silence, he voiced his opinion in no more than a few aperçus. To some of those present for the first time it felt as if he had come to his conclusions in the manner of a mystic. 'In the final analysis', he might say, 'we see only what we are ready to see, what we have been taught to see. We eliminate and ignore everything that is not part of our own prejudices.'

Once the last patient had left his office, he would put on his coat and top hat and leave for home. On his way out he was sometimes accosted by a patient begging for alms. Ensconced in his carriage, he would immediately begin to read, becoming so engrossed that his coachman reported that he often did not step down for several minutes after arriving back at L'hôtel de Varengeville on the Boulevard St Germain. Once lunch was over he would retire to his salon to recommence his studies. Sometimes he would work into the early hours of the morning catching up with the latest research published in German, English, Spanish and Italian as well as in French, and when his attention began to flag he would break off to do some sketches.

Charcot cut open cadavers in a renovated kitchen behind his consulting room. If his lancet revealed an alteration in the colour, volume or texture of the brain he drew a picture of the abnormality in a note-book and then included it in his post-mortem findings inserted in the patient's case records. He considered the autopsy to be an integral part of the clinical exami-nation, the last service one could offer to the patient and her family and an invaluable lesson in humility. His modus operandi is epitomised by the case of Luc, a woman who despite her clumsiness he employed as his domestic servant. Charcot observed that her hands shook when she carried a cup and saucer and that if her hands were motionless her head shook. Her unsteadi-ness gradually increased and when she could no longer work he arranged for her to be admitted to the hospice under his care. When she died, he performed a post-mortem examination and found numerous sclerotic plaques in the white matter of her brain and spinal cord, a finding that supported a condition he was in the course of differentiating from Parkinson's disease, which would later come to be called multiple sclerosis. His decision to employ Luc probably arose as much from his single-minded curiosity as his charity.

In 1882, a new amphitheatre was built in honour of Charcot's appointment as the first Professor of Diseases of the Nervous System and his weekly teaching sessions then became more structured but remained impromptu. Every Tuesday morning a large audience waited for him in silence and high expectation. At 9 a.m. he would enter the theatre with an entourage of clinical and laboratory chiefs, interns and visiting overseas fellows. He walked slowly across the dais to his chair, positioned to the left of the stage. The first patient would already be waiting in place. After a heavy pause he would begin to take their history:

Charcot: How old are you?
Patient: Thirty years.
Charcot: What do you do?
Patient: I am a tailor.
Charcot: Are you married?
Patient: My wife is dead.
Charcot: And when did your illness begin?
Patient: Thirteen months ago.
Charcot: And before that?
Patient: I had pain.
Charcot: What kind of pains?
Patient: Sudden stabbing pains in my legs that last at least twenty-four hours and during which the skin becomes sensitive. If I press hard on my legs it slightly relieves the pain.
Charcot: And during this time you were still walking and working?
Patient: Yes.

There were times when Charcot was unable to come to an immediate decision. On other occasions he was forced to admit he could not explain logically how he had arrived at his diagnosis. He would remind his audience that patients were allowed to have diseases that were rare and might even suffer from maladies that had not yet been identified. In the early stages of nervous disease an incomplete clinical presentation was usual, but this did not mean that a diagnosis could not be suspected. When there was uncertainty, it was best to describe exactly what one had heard and seen without prejudice and leave it at that.

Charcot was aware of his gift of seeing things in a flash, and to assist his audience he amplified his observations with memorable verbal descriptions. He also made drawings in chalk on the blackboard, showed lantern slides and temperature charts, and prepared posters and plaster casts to embellish his demonstration. An example of his ability to recount clearly what he had heard or seen is provided in this observation of the speech of a patient with multiple sclerosis:

There is a symptom more frequently found than nystagmus . . . and this is a peculiar difficulty in enunciation . . . The affected person speaks in a slow drawling manner and sometimes almost unintelligibly. It seems as if the tongue has become 'too thick', and the delivery recalls that of an individual suffering from incipient intoxication. A closer examination shows that the words are as if measured or scanned, there is a pause after every syllable, and the syllables themselves are pronounced slowly.

For some of his lessons, his clinical assistants would be asked to bring three or four patients into the amphitheatre at the same time. These people often looked completely different from one another but he knew, from his pathological work, that they represented different stages, or biological variations, of the same disease entity. If an example of a particular syndrome was not available for his presentation, he would imitate or pantomime an abnormal gait or a particular form of facial tic in order to embroider his description. His method owed little to inference or analysis but demanded extraordinary patience and a continuity of observation. In moments of reflection he would tell his disciples that he was nothing more than a photographer, but at the same time he was very aware of the limitations of static imagery and knew that pictures required captions, explanations and sequential categorisation for their clinical interpretation. Without his skill in focusing the camera's gaze, and the exactness of his accompanying written descriptions, the fading daguerreotypes, preserved in the hospital's iconography, would now be uninterpretable. Charcot's observations were far more than textbook accounts or snapshots of poorly people lying in bed: instead each seemed like a tableau of a life imprinted on an autobiography.

Although he emphasised that attentive listening and astute observation were essential to his method he also told his pupils that occasionally a coup d'oeil was all that was necessary to make a confident diagnosis. In one of his Tuesday lectures devoted to Parkinson's disease he said: 'I have seen such patients everywhere on the streets of Rome, of Amsterdam, in Spain, it is always the same picture: they can be identified from afar, you do not need a medical history.'

His teaching sessions left indelible pictures in the minds of his assistants, which no amount of private study could ever hope to replicate. Sigmund Freud, who spent the winter of 1885–86 as a visitor in Charcot's service, later wrote that he remembered coming out of one of these lessons fully sated with Charcot's words ringing in his ears, as if he was leaving Notre Dame with a new idea of perfection.

The entrance of L'Hôpital de la Salpêtrière was guarded by a majestic greystone cuboid with narrow windows and four turreted chimneys. I walked through its arched porch and down the long path that led to the first line of hospital buildings. Beyond the Mazarin gate stood the cruciform chapel of Saint-Louis, with its iconic domed roof, four naves and bleached walls. As I continued on down a footpath bordered by lindens and plane trees that formed one side of a large rectangular garden, the doleful peal of the church bells broke the leaden silence. I then turned left into Rue de la Lingerie and directly in front of me was La Force, the former prison with its inner courtyards named after Manon Lescaut and the September Massacres, where prostitutes and heretics had been contained before their deportation to Canada and Louisiana. After a few more minutes I arrived at a brutalist faded edifice that smelt of feline ammonia. I climbed the stone steps, opened the glass door and walked down a narrow passage lined with offices. At the end of the corridor was a lower hallway that ran at a right angle and led to the clinics. I took the lift up to the ward.

In the nurses office, over a breakfast of croissants and coffee, I was introduced to my new colleagues. Once the pleasantries were over discussion returned to the previous night's medical 'take' and specifically to an alcoholic, who had been admitted with amnesia due to acute Korsakoff's syndrome. After about half an hour François Lhermitte, the *chef de service*, arrived. He had a bulging cranium and wore his buttoned-up white coat with the collar upturned. His glasses seemed to enhance the twinkling inquisitiveness of his eyes as he looked at me as if I was a specimen from an alien world. He began by talking about a recently published paper in *Revue Neurologique* describing a group of people with focal damage to the globus pallidus who had profound mental inertia and slowness of thinking but without evidence of amnesia or dementia. I knew that he had a particular interest in behavioural disorders linked to frontal lobe disease and that he was also very exercised over whether thought was possible without words. His father, Jean Lhermitte, had preceded him on the staff of the hospital, and was best remembered in England and the United States of America for his description of an unusual symptom, occasionally reported by people with multiple sclerosis. In May 1924 he had reported the case of Madame D, a cashier who had come to see him at La Salpêtrière complaining of progressive loss of vision in one eye. She had told him that she had also noticed that whenever she lowered her neck a shock-like sensation occurred in her nape that spread down her back as far as her feet. The feeling was so unpleasant that in the last few months she had been unable to pick up objects from the ground unless she consciously avoided flexing her head. Lhermitte speculated in his article that the phenomenon was due to loss of insulation of the nerve fibres in the dorsal columns of the spinal cord leading to a short circuit each time the neck was inclined.

As we left the office to start the ward round Lhermitte whispered to his chief assistant: '*Ne me dis rien.*' On arriving at the bedside he asked the first patient what was troubling her, and after he had learned she was unsteady on her feet, how long she had been ill and then about any traumatic events that had occurred around the time of her first symptoms. He then enquired whether anyone else in the family had experienced unsteadiness and when she replied in the negative he seemed reluctant to accept this on face value. After further questioning he managed to extract from her that an uncle, who she had not seen for some years, was now apparently confined to a wheelchair.

His examination began by asking her to get out of bed and stand motionless with her eyes first open and then closed while one of his assistants stood guard in case she toppled over. The fact that she had not lost balance on closing her eyes told him that her ataxia was unlikely to be due to impairment of awareness of the position and movement of her body in space. He then asked her to walk up and down in the corridor outside her room commenting to us that her gait was lurching and broad-based. Next he asked her to try to walk with the toes of her back foot touching the heel of her front foot, a test commonly used by the police when trying to determine whether a motorist is intoxicated. When she attempted this she immediately toppled over to her left. He then asked her to pronate and supinate her outstretched hands with the elbows bent as fast as possible, which she could only do in a slow and jerky fashion. Finally he drew our attention to jerky nystagmus when she followed his finger with her eyes to the left or right. When we had left the bedside and returned to the corridor he told us he was certain that she had a hereditary cerebellar ataxia, a genetically heterogeneous group of disorders characterised by clumsiness of the hands, a slurred, scanning speech and an uncoordinated gait. As we moved on to see the next patient he smirked at one of his assistants and said: 'As soon as I saw all those different types of cigarette butt in her ashtray, I knew she must be an interesting case.'

Over time I realised that it was relatively unusual

for Lhermitte to carry out a focused neurological examination of the sort I had just witnessed. Particularly when dealing with a disorder of higher cerebral function his approach was often just to listen, observing the body language and analysing every move the patient made with endless fascination. He was a great impresario and his brio, insatiable curiosity and innovative ways of thinking about neurology would leave a lasting impression on me.

One day in La Salle Guillain, he took off his glasses and put them in the palm of his outstretched hand. Without a word the patient reached out for them and put them on over his own glasses. When asked to explain his conduct, the patient replied: 'Monsieur you gave it to me, so I thought I had to use it.' Lhermitte replied that nothing was expected and proceeded to hold out a comb. The man took it and ran it several times through his hair. Lhermitte turned triumphantly to his assistants and said, 'Have you seen? Did you see it?' None of us had an explanation for the patient's bizarre behaviour, although I remember wondering at the time whether subtle persuasion might have been used to induce it.

In those first few months I got into the routine of seeing patients on the wards, attending the occasional clinic and relishing the badinage that occurred over lunch in *la salle de garde*. My French contemporaries seemed to be more intuitive and observant and some of the signs we elicited had indelible romantic names like *le signe de la sonnette* (the doorbell sign), *l'epreuve de marionette* (the hand puppet test) and *la danse des tendons* (the dance of the tendons). Their clinical descriptions reminded me at times of extracts from Maupassant, Zola and Huysmans. Lhermitte often failed to show up for his ward round but the interns told me that he kept them on their toes by arriving unannounced at Saturday lunchtime just as they were about to go home, when he would demand that they stay on and show him an interesting patient. In his absence the *chef de clinique* led the round and before arriving at a final working diagnosis would always act as his own promoter and devil's advocate, thinking aloud and revising his views as more data was gathered. In arriving at a decision on what treatment to recommend what was more useful than evidence from multicentre drug trials with multiple exclusion criteria, was clinical nous and experience and a discussion of the social circumstances, occupation, family history, religion and hobbies of the sick person. Masterly inactivity and gentle medicine that I had often witnessed in London were culturally unacceptable in France. Another difference was that patients in France carried with them their own test results, many of which had been carried out in the private sector and which they expected to be reviewed.

Charcot's name was never mentioned by Lhermitte or his juniors: I assumed his pre-eminence was taken for granted. I was told by one of my new colleagues that Charcot's son, Jean-Baptiste, who had become a polar explorer after graduating in medicine, was now more widely remembered in France. With a Gallic shrug the *chef de clinique* told me that Charcot had dinted his reputation by his theatrical showmanship and use of hypnotism to treat hysteria. Charcot had left no confessions or personal memories to help me know what he was really like. Now I understood more about his ability to notice I wanted to understand from where his tremendous energy had sprung and how a taciturn family man not given to dangerous passions had ended up as a circus ringmaster. Sometimes as I strolled past the pharmacy where his consulting room had once stood or along the path next to the run-down chalets that remained from Charcot's day I sensed he was almost in touching distance. But if I was to learn more about him I needed to read what those who knew him had written but be equally wary of the Judas Iscariots, like Léon Daudet and Axel Munthe, and the honeyed betrayals of 'La Charcoterie'.

From Georges Guillain's biography, and the intimate reflections of Charcot's assistants Alexandre-Achille Souques, Henri Meige and Pierre Marie, I learned that Charcot had presided over his department with the authority of Napoléon. He had an abhorrence of sloppiness and imprecision and expected the same high standards in his assistants that he set for himself. In 1868 he had written: 'The scepticism of the human mind is a soft pillow for lazy heads; but in the epoch we are living it is no longer the time to fall asleep.'

When he was nettled, anger would flash in his eyes and his voice would become mordant and imperious. Colleagues from outside considered him aloof and disdainful and he was renowned for bearing lasting grudges against those who challenged his authority. But to his trusted disciples he was like a father, unwavering in his patronage and generous in his recognition of their achievements. Occasionally he would invite them to Les Folies Bergère but always leave discreetly before the dancing girls came on.

Away from work he was a different man altogether: affable, liberated and relaxed. At his Tuesday soirées, where any talk of medicine was forbidden, he and his family provided impeccable hospitality for some of Paris's greatest philosophers, artists, physicians and writers. To those fortunate enough to be present it seemed as though he radiated an interest in every topic of conversation. He was vehemently opposed to hunting and bullfighting and had a sign over his consulting room door saying: 'You will find no dog laboratory here'. Among his menagerie of pets were two dogs called Carlo and Sigurd, a donkey called Saladin, a pet monkey called Rosalie, who was allowed to run free in the dining room, and a macaw called Kiri. His natural quietude and love of animals led him to an affinity with the Buddha. From what I had gleaned I concluded that even if he had not been his carriage-maker father's chosen son, destined for academic greatness, he would have become famous throughout France for the elegance and artistry of his own coach design.

In his highly impressionistic memoir *The Story of San Michele* (1929) Axel Munthe wrote:

Charcot for instance was almost uncanny in the way he went straight to the root of the evil, often apparently only after a rapid glance at the patient from his cold eagle eyes. During the last years of his life maybe he relied too much upon his eye, the examination of his patients was often far too rapid and superficial.

It seemed to me that rather than having aquiline telescopic vision, Charcot glided between eye and brain like an African grey parrot. In the Brouillet salon print outside the library, Charcot seems to be observing his patient Blanche Wittmann out of the corner of one eye and the world at large with the other. In his studies on hysteria Charcot took the same unprejudiced observational approach that he had used with so much success in organic nervous disorders but in his last years before his death he accepted that it was a different beast and due to a psychic or physiological dysfunction in as yet unknown regions of the brain. He was also the first to recognise that hysteria was not confined to the female sex:

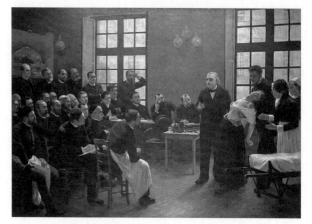

A Clinical Lesson at the Salpêtrière (1887)
by André Brouillet, which shows neurologist Jean-Martin
Charcot demonstrating hysteria in a hypnotised patient,
Blanche Wittmann.

For many years I walked through my wards like a blind man, never seeing hysteria in working men not because it was not there, after all it is not uncommon but because I did not know how to look at things. Only over the last six years have I really learned to see it.

After I had been in Paris for almost a year and learned as much as I could about Charcot from the French literature, I learned that my chief's grandfather, Léon Augustin Lhermitte, had been a naturalist painter who had focused on rustic scenes depicting peasants at work. When he had been asked by Van Gogh to reveal his technique he had said:

After I have caught sight of a man handling his scythe expertly I am not going to let him go. I will spend two or three hours in his tracks following his every step. I will watch him closely. I will watch him from afar and strive to apprehend the rhythm and pace of the movement.

François Lhermitte had added a holistic dimension to his clinical method, but like his grandfather and Charcot he too observed life through the prism of art. Charcot's shadow danced over every clinical discussion and pathological examination at the hospital and as a consequence there was no need for his illustrious successors to keep mentioning his name. After lunch I would walk the short distance from the hospital to the Garden of Plants and there vanish into the immensity of its prettiness. Immersed in the beauty of its hothouses and rose gardens I developed a technique of focusing just on whites, then on yellows, and seeing how the colour jumped out from the herbaceous borders. Behind a veil of pines I caught glimpses of the mechanised city veiled in a violet haze. Charcot was able to listen to nervous diseases with his eyes in the same way a botanist observed the germination of buried seeds and the rupture of buds. Looking back I remember these moments as some of the happiest of my life. I felt as if I had been released from gravity and time and suffused with a deep peace.

Jean-Martin Charcot had ushered me to a front row seat

in the stalls for an unequalled dramatic performance and taught me that art imitates life, but never quite measures up to it. If I was to try to copy his method I needed to raise my brow, suppress my blink, dilate my pupils and hold each patient in fixed view. To visualise afresh I needed to return to the panoramic floodlight curiosity of childhood – to train myself to recognise and remember the external signs that together are required for the coherent expression of each clinical syndrome. Keeping my eyes wide open would involve perceiving what was absent, as well as recognising what was in plain sight in front of my nose.

Paris had begun to awaken. Its streets no longer seemed shabby and full of cowed people devoid of gaiety. I started to closely observe others before they saw me and zoom in and out on their gestures, postures and facial expressions. With my exploding turquoise ticket I could now see everything without being seen and was able to transform time into space. My Métro plan mapped each new nervous disease to a particular subterranean beach. After my first ever sighting Gilles de la Tourette syndrome was connected to Glacière, and on Ligne 1 at Pont de Neuilly I diagnosed the inappropriate winking of a bureaucrat as hemifacial spasm. I was frequenting platforms that smelled of Parma Violets and coming out through iron turnstiles that connected me to La Belle Époque.

On one of my many return visits to Paris I learned that Lhermitte had taken his research out of the clinic and the laboratory and into the world at large. In a presentation he had recently delivered to La Société Française de Neurologie on 3 December 1981 he had startled the audience when, after rising to the podium, without a word of explanation he had left it and walked briskly up to the middle of the auditorium, where he had then made his way along one of the rows holding out his hand to each member of the audience. Miracle of miracles all of them spontaneously shook his hand. His aim was to show that the handshake is irresistible and can be interpreted as a culturally dependent gesture of peace. He then showed a film of several patients with frontal lobe lesions, one of whom was a former nurse that he had taken to his apartment in the Rue de Tournon and who, on seeing the room laid out like a consulting room without instruction auscultated Lhermitte's chest, then picked up a needle and syringe from a table and injected him in the buttocks. His loyal assistants, some of whom I knew well, had feared for his reputation, while longstanding colleagues and adversaries all questioned his sanity. Several years later this work was published with an accompanying glowing editorial in the well-respected American journal *Annals of Neurology*. In his paper, Lhermitte proposed that the occurrence of utilisation and imitation behaviour in people with frontal lobe damage had led him to conclude that one of the purposes of the prefrontal cortex was to allow human beings to escape from a dependency on their immediate environment and in the course of their evolution it had permitted them to venture down from the trees. His article was also notable for the fact that it was the first and only time in the history of neurology that an author's buttocks had been displayed for posterity in a published illustration. The abnormal behaviour he had demonstrated in the patient in La Salle Guillain all those years ago and which we had failed to understand now became a routine bedside test to evaluate prefrontal lobe dysfunction, analogous to the Babinski sign that had been used for a century to detect damage to the central motor pathways in the brain and spinal cord.

After my journeyman year in Paris, my powers of inspection improved greatly. Now as I listened to patients' narratives, I scrutinised their faces. I looked for freezing of spontaneous expression, asymmetry of the nasolabial folds, drooping of the eyelids and squints, premature baldness, xanthelasma, cataracts or operation scars. I made a conscious note of any involuntary jerking, trembling or spasms or unusual body or limb postures. If the patient had epilepsy I would search the skin for *café au lait* spots, sebaceous adenomas, shagreen patches and port wine stains. I always checked the nails, the conjunctiva and the cornea. I would then feel the skin of each hand and foot for regional warmth or coldness. In a patient with Cushing's syndrome I pinched up a thin fold of skin between my fingers, and in an elderly woman with scleroderma

I was able to feel that the skin was abnormally tight and adherent. In my future clinical narratives I aimed to convey the panoply of neurological phenomena with the directness and precision of a Métro line. The lives of my patients and the questions they asked me would from now on become the focus of my fieldwork. I was finally convinced I was in the right job.

– This Is the Ritual –

The nervous system is almost entirely inaccessible to the naked eye, but through the study of external signs it is possible to localise areas of damage and make diagnoses that sometimes have not been considered after the medical interview. The scheme that I was taught was perfected by the Dublin-born British neurologist Dr Gordon Holmes in the years between the two World Wars. By deploying the anatomo-clinical method first used by Laennec and then Charcot he was able to validate his examination technique and elevate the neurological examination to a greater level of precision. Holmes taught the 'how' of symptomatology and the functional importance of physical signs.

MacDonald Critchley told me of Holmes' exacting and exorbitant demands on his junior staff. During his own time as Holmes' house physician, Critchley had been expected to be on duty twenty-four hours a day, look up obscure references for his chief and when one of Holmes' patients had died suddenly he had been dispatched to a remote farmstead in rural Essex and instructed to perform an autopsy on the kitchen table.

Gordon Holmes' ward rounds were carried out behind locked doors at the National Hospital and also at Charing Cross Hospital, which was situated then in Agar Street, just off the Strand. His devoted nursing staff saw to it that his patients remained stock-still and only opened their mouths when spoken to. With his lowered eyebrows and strigine gaze he punctiliously examined each of them from top to toe, irrespective of whether a diagnosis had already been established. If there were incongruities in his findings he would break away and walk to the window, standing there silently for several minutes. On his return to the bedside he would start afresh, recapitulating the clinical history with the patient and double-checking the validity of any signs that didn't fit. His infallible method hinged on practised, organised common sense. At the end of the ward round that usually lasted several hours his staff were exhausted whereas he appeared as fresh as a daisy. Holmes wrote that the student of neurology must be equipped with an intellectual honesty and independence that refuses to submit to authority or be dominated by preconception. If the neurological examination was to be of value it needed to be conducted with the discipline of a laboratory experiment.

Anecdotes about the Victorian and Edwardian founding fathers of neurology formed a very important part of my education. I agreed instinctively with Holmes that in situations where lives were at stake, there was no place for lackadaisical dilettantism. Far from filling me with horror, his dedicated and modest search for the truth spurred me on. I admired the fact that he had been able to achieve so much without a medical department or even an office and his professionalism inspired me to strive for greater precision in my own clinical method.

A few months into my specialist training at University College Hospital in 1975 I was bleeped by one of the nurses to say that a patient had been admitted as an emergency and that her husband wanted to see me. When I drew back the curtains, a small man in his forties with gimlet eyes wearing a woolly pullover was sitting in the bedside chair. Before I had time to introduce myself he got up and asked me how long his wife would have to be in hospital. He then launched into an account of the events that had taken place earlier that day in the outpatient department across the road in Cecil Fleming House on Grafton Way:

When we were telling Dr Stern what was wrong with Maureen he hardly said a 'dicky bird'. He then asked the missus to get undressed and lie on a couch behind a screen. After a few minutes he appeared with a student. First he asked her to take sevens away from one hundred as if she was training for a darts match. Next off, she had to close her eyes and sniff some coffee in a glass tube. He then got her to remember a name and address, and while she was doing that he shone a torch in her eyes. I then saw her following his moving finger with her gaze. Next up he asked her to screw her eyes up as if there were soap in 'em and he pushed a wooden stick down her throat. She then had to push and pull as hard as she could against his hands until she was ready to drop. He then lifted up the blanket and had a good look at her 'pins', made her knee jump with his cosh and her ankle judder by yanking her foot towards her. He then pricked her bottom, moved her big toe up and down and asked her if she could feel the vibrations of his tuning fork in her toes.

At this point Maureen finally managed to get a word in and said to me: 'Dr Stern's the business, enny doc?' Maureen was full of admiration for my chief and his thoroughness but the fact that her husband had been so anxious to get off his chest what he had witnessed in the clinic made me think a bit more about a protocol I had always taken for granted. If I wanted patients to fully participate in the unfolding drama of the physical examination it was probably wise to explain what each manoeuvre I carried out would involve and the reason behind doing it.

Maureen told me she had low back pain which was worse when she was lying down when it radiated round her abdomen in a tight band, and that she had started to trip up inexplicably when walking. When I flexed her right knee there was an initial catch reminiscent of the opening of the blade of a penknife. She was also unable to straighten her bent right knee against resistance or flex her right hip against the force of my hand. When I scratched the outer aspect of her sole with an orange stick, her right big toe turned upwards, a sign indicative of damage to the descending corticospinal tract and attributed to the French neurologist Joseph

Babinski. These abnormalities on examination all pointed to an injury somewhere in the motor pathway that transmitted commands from her brain down the spinal cord to her legs and ruled out the possibility that her symptoms were due to damage to her nerve roots, peripheral nerves or muscles. I next tested her sensory system and found that she could not feel pain or appreciate hot and cold sensations in her left leg and the lower abdomen to the level of her umbilicus. When considered in conjunction with the abnormalities of the motor system these findings allowed me to locate her problem with reasonable certainty to the lower part of the thoracic spinal cord. A few days later myelography, in which dye is injected through a lumbar puncture needle into the spinal canal, confirmed that Maureen had a space-occupying lesion at the level of the tenth thoracic vertebra. Mr Bernard Harries, the neurosurgeon, successfully removed a tumour the size of a cherry that had started to press on the right side of the spinal cord. A sample from the lump was stained, and a thin section of the tissue examined under the microscope revealing it to be a benign neoplasm called a neurofibroma.

It was not uncommon for me as a registrar in neurology to spend two or more hours examining a patient. The testing of orientation, memory, language, arithmetic, executive function and perception took a minimum of half an hour and sometimes far longer when there was suspected pathology in the cerebral hemispheres. Sometimes I would need to complete my bedside cognitive evaluation in two stages to avoid the patient becoming tired and distractible. I would then test visual acuity with a Snellen chart, a large rectangular white card with a scale of letters printed in successively decreasing sizes, before taking the patient to a darkened room to look at the back of the eye with my ophthalmoscope. I plotted the visual fields by confrontation testing using a red hatpin brought into the field of vision from the margins. If I suspected inflammation of the optic nerve I would look carefully for a blind spot in the central field of vision known as a scotoma. Loss of colour vision in one eye revealed by the Ishihara plates was another abnormal sign that pointed to a diagnosis of optic neuritis. I would then systematically work my way downwards, examining each of the remaining eleven pairs of cranial nerves in turn before going on to assess tone, power and coordination in the arms and legs.

My first tendon hammer was given to me by a friend who had worked as a junior doctor at the National Hospital, Queen Square and had later decided to go into gastroenterology. It had a long, slender, tapering bamboo handle, surmounted by a deeply grooved sphere of bell-metal and a stout ring of India rubber let into the metal indentation to help cushion the blow. Once I had mastered the sharp, undamped wrist flick needed to make a tendon jump, my hammer transformed into a magic wand. Each time I struck the Achilles tendon I imagined a synchronous volley of electrical impulses travelling from the nerve endings in the muscle spindles up sensory nerves to the first sacral segment of the spinal cord where they connected through synapses with nerve fibres that connected with the calf muscles. Other nervous impulses that descended the spinal cord were firing away at the same time to activate antagonist muscles at the ankle so as to dampen the force of the jerk. I recorded the response to each tendon tap using a score that ranged from one minus for an absent jerk through one plus for normal up to three pluses if I considered the tendon reflex to be pathologically brisk. My tendon hammer allowed me to conduct an autopsy in life and imagine the invisible. I could not have taken more care of it if it had been a Stradivarius violin.

I would conclude by examining the sensory system, testing light touch with a wisp of cotton wool, pain with a pin, vibration sense with a tuning fork and joint position sense by asking the patient, with eyes closed, to detect the slightest movement I made in an upwards or downwards direction to the side of their middle finger and their big toe. In contrast to inspection, which relied entirely on observation, the examination of a patient required a feeling finger. There were also opportunities to use my ears. With my stethoscope I once heard the machinery murmur of a fistula over the eye and on another occasion the sound of a helicopter coming from the thigh of a patient who felt unsteady and shaky on standing. Audible clicks arising in the muscles of the Eustachian tube were diagnostic of a palatal tremor. Learning to read medical semiotics was allowing me to graduate from sympathetic conversation to accurate diagnosis. While my notes on a patient's particular medical history often resembled a treatise of literary realism, the examination findings possessed the objectivity of a chemistry experiment.

Depending on the patient's symptoms my teachers used an abbreviated examination technique to assist them in localising the lesion, a term used in medicine to indicate the site but not the cause of disease. When a patient complained of inexplicably dropping objects held in her right hand they might ask her to hold her hands out with the palms facing upwards and then close her eyes. If in the next few seconds the hand slowly and involuntarily pronated, that was sufficient to confirm their suspicion of subtle weakness. If, instead of a downward drift, they noticed a writhing of the fingers, they would next test joint position sense, looking for sensory ataxia. If, when they pushed down on her outstretched hands, there was an exaggerated upward rebound movement, they would then get her to touch her nose with her finger, looking for any sign of tremulousness as the finger approached the target that would suggest a problem with the cerebellum. They would then always watch the patient sit, stand and walk down the corridor. The company which each physical sign kept was always of importance when interpreting its significance. As well as making a note of these useful shortcuts, I also wrote down in my notebook 'smart handles' that would allow me to open a drawer with the answer inside; 'canaries' that were established harbingers of nervous disease and 'red flag' warnings of exclusion. I learned that an elderly man who has been referred with concerns over dementia and who turns up for an outpatient appointment under his own steam is much more likely to have depression or even a functional amnesia. Headache, fever and focal pain can precede the vesicular rash in shingles by up to two weeks. A woman with neurological symptoms wearing sunglasses may have photosensitivity due to a local ocular disorder or migraine but is more likely to have a psychogenic disorder. Despite their fallibility and lack of scientific scrutiny these 'rules of thumb', passed down from one generation of neurologists to the next, proved far more useful to me than retained textbook factual knowledge.

When I was concerned about shortcomings in my examination technique David Perkin, the senior registrar, always found the time to show me where I was going wrong. In my first week of neurology training at University College Hospital he had already recommended that I examine the patient before consulting the case notes. By doing it this way I would avoid the endemic problem of collective acquiescence among trainees known as The Emperor's New Clothes syndrome, and at the same time increase the chances of revealing something others had missed. He warned me against inventing physical signs in order to impress, and that in medicine errors of commission were as dangerous as errors of omission. Learning to examine a patient proficiently was not unlike learning French, and once I had mastered it exciting opportunities of discovery would open up.

One day I accompanied him to see a man with multiple sclerosis who had been admitted to the ward for a five-day course of intravenous corticosteroids. When David asked the patient to look to the left I noticed that the man's right eye did not move and remained looking straight ahead while at the same time some jerky rapid nystagmus was noticeable in the abducted left eye. He then asked the patient to focus on his finger as he brought it closer and closer. Both of the man's eyes converged normally, showing that the muscle that moved the right eye inwards could not be paralysed. This was the first time I had seen the physical sign known as an internuclear ophthalmoplegia. He then escorted the patient into a darkened side room and swung the beam of his pen torch from one pupil to the other at three-second intervals. I noted that every time the torchlight fell on the right eye the pupil constricted briskly, but when it moved over to the left eye there was a slightly delayed rebound dilatation. David told me that this indicated that the afferent arc of the light reflex was faulty. He went on to say that when an internuclear ophthalmoplegia and an afferent pupil defect occurred together in a young or middle-aged person the probability that the diagnosis was multiple sclerosis was high. What astonished me was that although the patient had no symptoms relating to his vision, David's examination had located lesions in the left optic nerve and the median longitudinal bundle, a group of crossed axons in the brainstem that connected the three cranial nerves involved in synchronous eye movement.

With constant practice I came to appreciate the wide variation in power and coordination that was present in healthy people. I developed strategies to help patients relax when I was trying to assess their muscle tone and I became more polished in tapping tendons. After almost missing marked muscle-wasting and weakness in the shoulder girdle of a young woman with muscular dystrophy whose only complaint was a difficulty in climbing stairs, I never forgot how important it was in any suspected case of neuromuscular disease to explain tactfully the absolute essential requirement of full exposure of the trunk and limbs. Contrary to my teaching at medical school I discovered through experience that the testing of sensation was more effective if the patient was not asked to close their eyes. The absence of a neurological sign could also be as informative as when it was present. For instance, in a patient complaining of lumbago and sciatica, if I found the ankle jerk to be intact, lumbar nerve root entrapment was less likely than if it were absent.

*

Once, after we had been to see a patient with visual hallucinations on the psychiatric ward at St Pancras Hospital, Dr Stern told me that his former boss in Newcastle, Henry Miller, had described psychiatry as 'neurology without physical signs'. He explained that Miller's adage had not meant to be derogatory but rather serve to encourage neurologists to embrace the social brain. The continuing conflict of paradigms that prevailed between neurology and psychiatry was emphasised to me one day when a young man was admitted. Having suddenly become paralysed at home, he complained that he felt as if his legs were no longer connected to his body. There was no past medical history of relevance and he denied any childhood traumas. On examination, his arms and legs were very weak, but all his reflexes were present and his appreciation of pain, touch, temperature, joint position and vibration sense were normal. When he was asked to voluntarily extend his right hip by pressing both heels down into the bed there was no movement, but when he was encouraged to flex his left hip against the resistance of my hand, his right hip extended involuntarily. This finding, known as Hoover's sign, pointed to probable psychogenic weakness and he was diagnosed with a motor conversion disorder. Although I had become aware of the limitations inherent in the neurological examination, this case seemed to reinforce how valuable it could be in allowing me to detect invisible lesions of the mind.

He was seen by a psychiatrist who interviewed

him on two separate occasions but could find no evidence of mental illness. Dr Stern told him that there was every chance that his exhausted nervous system would recover over time and he was treated with electrical stimulation, hypnotism and finally an injection of sodium amytal. The junior nurses doted on him and he had many visitors. During one of his daily physiotherapy sessions he sank like a stone to the bottom of the pool when he was left momentarily unsupported, and there were no reports of him moving during his sleep at night. After several months in the hospital, contractures started to develop in his swollen hands and feet.

There was no improvement in his paralysis and eventually he was transferred to a dingy and rather depressing long-stay rehabilitation ward in another hospital. A few weeks later I received a phone call from the registrar to say that he had almost completely recovered. When Dr Stern and I saw him again in the outpatient clinic nearly a year after his paralysis he was walking without any form of assistance and he told us that he was confident that he would now fully recover. The only possible trigger for his catastrophic illness we were ever able to find was that shortly before the onset of his paralysis he had narrowly failed to qualify for the British Olympic Judo Team.

The physical examination is neither outdated nor obsolete and it is far more efficient in localising the site of the neurological problem than any single machine. If the big toe goes up when I scrape the outer sole I can say with absolute conviction that the pathway carrying impulses from the motor cortex on the contralateral side of the brain down to the anterior horn cells of the spinal cord is disinhibited. The realisation that a single genetic mutation can present very differently even in members of the same family has given a new impetus to Gordon Holmes' scheme. Advances in rehabilitation for stroke and head injury and the emergence of new therapies for diseases for which there was no treatment have also reinforced the need for a repeated systematic semi-quantitative examination in assessing change. Without a detailed physical examination the interpretation of a patient's symptoms in relation to their impact on behaviour and habits also becomes less meaningful.

Even if the neurological examination were to become one day redundant, I would still lay on hands during the medical consultation. The intimate bond of touch, as part of the diagnostic process, changes the dynamic between patient and doctor forever, and it is a shame that psychiatrists have been forced for whatever reason to forego it. It also serves as a transcendent comforting force that promotes trust and reduces loneliness, anxiety and despair. Touch comes before words and is the first and last language. It is an essential constituent of healing and another way of listening that never lies.

– The Lost Soul of Neurology –

Neurology is a young medical speciality whose origins can be traced back to the efforts of a few enlightened physicians who believed that the brain was the organ of the mind and that localisation of symptoms could be achieved by meticulous clinical and pathological study. These doctors, many of whom worked in mental asylums in the middle of the nineteenth century, no longer considered epilepsy to be a supernatural spiritual disorder controlled by the moon, but the result of a focus of irritation in the cerebral hemispheres. They viewed autopsies as an extension of the clinical diagnostic process and any disorder that could not be positively identified after the pathological examination was referred to as a neurosis.

Over time these physicians with a special interest in the study of nervous diseases distanced themselves from the 'mad doctors' known as alienists who were little more than custodians of the mentally ill. An adherent to this anatomo-clinical approach was Sigmund Freud, who began his article published in the *Wiener Medizinische Wochenschrift* as follows: 'On January 17, 1884, a sixteen-year-old shoemaker apprentice was admitted bleeding profusely from the gums and showed multiple rose-red punctiform haemorrhages on the lower legs.' Freud then goes on to describe in great detail his serial examinations of the boy's delayed neurological deterioration that would lead to his death. A paralysis of eye movement, pin-point pupils, decorticate rigidity of the neck and limbs and Cheyne-Stokes breathing ('Between one group of breaths and the next there are pauses of fourteen to fifteen seconds') were all described in his report. The post-mortem examination confirmed that there had been numerous small bleeds into the brain as a result of scurvy leading to a herniation of the cerebral hemispheres. In his conclusion he made the point that by examining the boy regularly he had been able to follow the extent of the bleeding in the brain and predict his eventual demise.

A year later Freud left Vienna to spend a few months studying under Jean-Martin Charcot in Paris. When Freud arrived at La Salpêtrière Charcot's research on hysteria was in full swing, and his new chief was reluctantly being forced to concede, at least in private, that however hard one looked at the brain of a hysteric under the microscope the cause of the symptoms remained hidden from view. Freud was intrigued by what he had seen, and on his return to Vienna he perfected an unphysiological method called free association where his neurotic patients were encouraged to talk freely without censure about whatever ideas or memories occurred to them. Freud hoped that in the same way noticing had allowed Charcot to define organic nervous disease, attentive listening would enable him to understand the pathology of mental illness. As part of his method he also interpreted patients' dreams with the purpose of unearthing deep-seated emotional traumas and unconscious wish fulfilment. The growth in popularity of psychoanalysis with the reification of Freudian dogma in the first half of the twentieth century contributed to a growing split between doctors who studied diseases of the brain in hospitals and those who studied disorders of the mind in offices. Analysts restricted their observations to the interpretation of gestures as they listened and then interpreted their patients' stories. Physical signs frequently observed in psychiatric hospitals and described by physicians at the end of the nineteenth century – such as catalepsy, *gegenhalten* and verbigeration – were now looked upon as ambiguous approximations and non-specific symbols, rather than indicators of higher cerebral dysfunction.

Diseases of the nervous system can humiliate in a way that cancer or heart disease never do. Neurological symptoms are strange, subtle and often unpredictable, and even a tiny injury to a very small part of the brain can leave a person changed forever. In a single moment a stroke can take away the ability to walk and converse, and Alzheimer's disease eventually removes any sense of a future or a past. A full recovery may occur after an attack of multiple sclerosis that has caused painful loss of vision in one eye, but be followed inexplicably

– months or years later – by a relapse that leads to permanent unsteadiness, anaesthesia in the legs and incontinence of urine. Creeping paralysis can take away an individual's ability to swallow, move, breathe and talk, even while leaving the mind intact. Victims of the shaking palsy describe feelings as if they are walking in treacle and talking from behind a mask. Fits feel like the unpredictable intrusion of an alien power or a banshee screeching in pain. The horrible uniqueness of each of these devastating maladies is what makes neurology such an emotionally exacting speciality.

Early in my career I became aware that there were different types of neurologists. Most behaved like bumble bees, gathering pollen from the flowers of the field, and transforming and digesting it through their own deductive powers into a clinical diagnosis. A few conducted themselves like spiders, weaving ideas from their own substance, while the rest resembled ants, constantly collecting data to disprove theories for the common good. What united them all was an antipathy towards psychiatry. What separated psychiatry from neurology and all of science was that not only could its beliefs, theories and to a large extent its practice not be questioned but that it was forbidden to even challenge that they could not be questioned. Its self-contained syndicate had divorced itself from human beings and resisted all substantive challenges to its code of practice as being anti-psychiatry. By the nineteen seventies, when psychiatry had started to return to its medical roots and pills were being used to reset chemical messenger balance in the brain, it seemed even more divorced from reality. Things had undergone a further change for the worse and there were now very few specialists in psychological medicine interested in the socio-anthropological aspects of human life and experience, or the cultural aspects of behaviour.

William Gooddy, one of my first teachers at University College Hospital, told me over coffee and Bourbon biscuits in the day room how Thomas Willis was the bee, spider and ant in one man. Willis had opened skulls in the back rooms of inns in order to locate the mind, likening the brain to a kingdom of provinces and villages, irrigated by rivulets of blood, and drained by ventricles. The supreme commands were discharged through animal spirits in the cranial nerves that sparked involuntary muscular movements 'like the explosion of gunpowder'. It was the disembodied soul that provided Man with higher thought, free will and judgement and a second material 'soul of brutes' that was responsible for the rhythms of respiration, peristalsis and the pumping of the heart. Willis wrote that 'the problem of neurology is to understand man himself'. He believed that some of the nervous conditions he described in his medical casebook were due to disorders of chemical fermentation within the brain's alembic.

Thomas Willis considered empathy to be a variant of self-pity and that it could be simulated. Gooddy too believed that a trainee who claimed to feel a sharp stab in his back when he performed a lumbar puncture was unlikely to survive the rigours of clinical practice for very long. A doctor could never know what it was like to experience the terror of losing one's mind. He told us that after an insult to the brain, the normal cycles of nervous activity were blocked and however much healing occurred the affected person would never be the same again. It was not enough simply to recognise a patient's distress and suffering; what was important for a physician was to have the courage and competence to do something about it. When the teaching round was over, I walked with him past the nursing bay and through the ward. As we arrived at the office at the top of the stairs, he turned to me and said: 'Lees, neurology is deadly serious but it must also be full of soul.'

Growing up in St Helens I had been imbued with soulfulness tempered with common sense and having just returned from a year in Paris it was easy for me to take my teacher's comment at face value. As a child I had looked down my throat with a torch to see if I could spot my ethereal essence in the mirror and my mother had told me that even objects could come to life if their souls were awakened. I now believed that my soul was not located in the lower brainstem but was composed of the sum of all my neuronal connections. My soul possessed a loving, reverberating energy that had the power to light up a room and the more I linked my brain's signature with life, the more my passion would help me open the door to health. It was comparable to energy or parallel universes and went way beyond wonder drugs or brain surgery.

I felt fortunate to have come into contact early in my career with two master storytellers: both Dr Gooddy and Dr Stern brought their experience, their art and their lives, to the bedside and taught me to think independently. They inspired me to crawl through gaps in the barbed wire fence that divides art from science and dig a hole under the high wall that had sprung up between hospital and university. Although each subscribed to the view that psychiatry was a guild profession distinct from the rest of medicine with not a single validated clinical test, they fed my curiosity to explore the exciting but menacing border that lay between it and neurology.

Both my teachers stressed the importance of writing in plain English and warned against what Michael O'Donnell, one of medicine's best writers, would later call the 'decorated municipal gothic' style, which he defined as 'long, tortuous, opaque, uninteresting with a built-in quality of unreadability'. Gooddy described baroque words like dysdiadochokinesia and akathisia which had a strong foothold in neurology as snakes that dragged their ungainly lengths across the page. Many of the disorders they taught me about have since received different names: Charcot-Marie-Tooth disease has become hereditary and sensory neuropathy type 1 and Bell's palsy has become idiopathic facial paralysis. These revisions sometimes reflected the acquisition of new knowledge but were more often driven by an attempt to be more scientifically precise. Some have been an improvement, like the use of 'stroke' instead of 'cerebrovascular accident', but others like 'complex partial seizures' instead of 'temporal lobe epilepsy' are less satisfactory. Without context a patient cannot understand why the episodes of disordered consciousness she is experiencing are complex or partial.

The use of eponyms in medicine continues to polarise opinion. Much has been written about their limitations, but it cannot be denied that many have usefully stood the test of time. They are succinct and memorable and when used in moderation add lustre and colour. As a medical student they increased my curiosity about the people behind the names and led to a habit that I have continued during my career of going back to the seminal accounts of a disease even when it was described in the distant past. Gilles de la Tourette syndrome is a beautiful name for a distressing disorder, which perhaps if it had been forced to carry the prosaic label of chronic multiple tics with abnormal vocalisations forever might still not have achieved public recognition. Some eponyms like Parkinson's and Alzheimer's have survived unscathed for more than a century while others, such as Morvan's fibrillary chorea, are now obsolete. Most, however, are rightly in flux such as mongolism which became Down's syndrome and then Down syndrome and perhaps will become Trisomy 21. Briquet's syndrome briefly succeeded hysteria but has now been replaced by somatic symptom disorder or functional neurological disorder and Binswanger's disease is gradually losing out to the unwieldy subcortical leukoencephalopathy. La maladie de Steinert is restricted to the Francophone world while in Germany the same condition of myotonic dystrophy is sometimes referred to as Curschmann-Steinert-Syndrom.

Some scientifically minded doctors dislike eponyms and toponyms on the grounds that they tell one nothing about the pathophysiology of the disease. The opponents also argue that they have the potential to vilify a place such as Marburg or glorify wicked doctors, like Julius Hallervorden, whose soul had been corrupted by Nazism. But sometimes they avoid stigma, as in Hansen's disease not leprosy, Angelman's syndrome not happy puppet syndrome, and some like Hartnup disease even commemorate patients. Familial British dementia, multiple system atrophy, SCA7 and C9orf72 are some of the awkward labels that have been adopted by committee with scant thought for the patients who have to bear them, or their families.

While I have a soft spot for eponyms, I dislike abbreviations. How many doctors outside the narrow field of movement disorders for example know that SWEDDS stands for 'scans without evidence of dopaminergic deficit'? Abbreviations have different meanings for different people even within the separate specialities of medicine. PSP, used in medicine to save breath instead of progressive supranuclear palsy means PlayStation Portable to a teenager and Payment Service Provider to a businessman. I agree with George Bernard Shaw who, in his play *The Doctor's Dilemma*, included abbreviations amongst his list of conspiracies used by the professions to acquire prestige, power and wealth.

Acronyms can be just as irritating but sometimes redeem themselves by being amusing, like VOMIT (victims of modern imaging technology), literary like POEMS (polyneuropathy, organomegaly, endocrinopathy and monoclonal gammopathies) or romantic like CLIPPERS (chronic lymphocytic inflammation with pontine perivascular enhancement responsive to steroids). A collection of more than 30,000 medical acronyms has been published on the internet. They are also used by doctors as a secret language to express the unspeakable truth about some of their patients.

Soulful neurology has realistic expectations that allow me to reduce the burden of suffering through my understanding of life as well as my scientific credentials. It embraces anecdote, cordial laughter and tacit knowledge but never lapses into sentimentality. It insists that mistakes in medicine are inevitable, but when they are admitted and taken to heart become future friends. It expects me to talk unhurriedly to patients as if they were my close relatives and to try to be kind and nuanced when forced to give bad news. It reminds me that neurological disorders can rupture aspirations and dreams and lead to frustration, loneliness and a profound sense of hopelessness. I see it as a branch of ecology that fuses the power of the neurological examination with the rich lived experience of the patient and which frees me to believe in happy accidents, the possibility of miracles and the healing power of faith.

– Words –

My seven years of postgraduate training came down to contact with people who took an interest in me. The intersections were always haphazard, but when they occurred, I took advantage of my good fortune. By the time I was appointed a consultant neurologist in 1982 I knew that listening was a more proactive and challenging skill than observation. Listening was different from hearing and only became of diagnostic value when it was combined with the skill to decipher a patient's utterances and then act upon them. Antennae, as well as ears, were sometimes needed to make sense of what was being said. Listening required patience, sensitivity and versatility and could only be mastered by constant practice. I learned to focus not just on the words but the rate of speech, the pause-to-speech ratio, the pitch, tone and volume of the voice, the gaps between each word, and the inflections as well as any accompanying gestures.

Nowadays, at the beginning of every consultation, I greet the patient in the waiting room with a professional smile and formally introduce myself. I remind the nurses and reception staff that I must not be interrupted and switch off my mobile phone. I ask the patient to sit opposite me and a little to my left. Family members or carers are seated further back so I can observe their reactions to the questions I address directly to the patient. I try to signal by my demeanour that I am both interested in what I am about to hear and that I have all the time in the world. I then start by asking the patient to tell me what has brought her to the hospital. I concentrate on the story as if I was listening to a riveting lecture and suspend all other frames of reference. I might nod to encourage, but I rarely interrupt. I work always on the assumption that I am being told the whole truth. Most patients stop talking after about five minutes, after which I ask a few open-ended questions that help to provide crucial additional diagnostic information.

Patients' stories are not always easy to listen to and are often harder to tell. If I am told: 'Doctor I am not feeling myself', I always take it very seriously. If I sense despair or a need for sympathy, I might say: 'I think it is incredible how brave you are and how you manage to do so much.'

No word is neutral. Humpty Dumpty says scornfully to Alice that when he uses a word it means just what he chooses it to mean, neither more nor less. In a similar vein, Joseph Conrad wrote that, 'Half the words we use have no meaning whatever and of the other half each man understands each word under the fashion of his own folly and conceit.' Each word is a living being with descendants, and words – like wells – can accommodate all manner of waters. When I am uncertain what a patient means when they use terms like numbness, weakness, giddiness or blackouts I may say something like 'Could you explain what you mean by a fit?' I then enquire about the past medical history. If I suspect a hereditary cause of the symptoms I may ask permission to talk to the accompanying family members in private. If the family history indicates siblings, parents or children who may be similarly affected, I ask if it is possible for them to attend with the patient at the follow-up visit so I can examine them, or whether the patient can try to obtain agreement for me to contact the doctor who is looking after the affected family member. I then ask what medicines, including those bought over the counter, are being taken and use this list as a cross-check for ongoing chronic complaints that may have been forgotten or not mentioned in the past medical history. If I suspect a tropical disease, I ask about recent travel.

All the time I am on the lookout for verbal and visual signals indicative of fear or worry. I pay attention to slips of the tongue or seemingly casual or flippant remarks. I ask questions like: 'Do you have any particular concerns about this?' or begin a question with: 'Oh, just one more thing.' I use brief silences to draw out hidden agendas. Sometimes I record the patient's exact description in quotes in the case notes: 'My face is split open and the bones feel as if they are shattering and the flesh is being scraped raw by red-hot claws.'

At the end I ask the family if they have anything further to add. A patient's recall of their medical history is often unreliable and the presence of relatives can be helpful, especially in the corroboration of dates and past medical events. Over time I have learned when to probe and when to leave alone and appreciate the value of short silences. The presenting complaint can often be totally unrelated to the real problem and I am always on the alert for an unspoken subtext that exposes the true other. Listening carefully to what the patient tells me gives me the diagnosis in seven out of every ten patients I see.

Arriving at a diagnosis involves matching the symptoms and their course with those of a recognised pattern that has been given a special name. Sherlock Holmes' methods of searching for clues were more effective than those of Inspector Lestrade, 'the best of the professionals' at the Metropolitan Police Force, because he knew, through his experience and imagination, which bits of the victim's narrative were important in helping him solve the case. Holmes avoided tunnel hearing, where he only listened to the specifics of the crime, and never allowed preconceptions to influence his detective work.

There are similarities between the way I try to obtain information and an interview conducted by the Criminal Investigation Department. A skilled detective understands the value of letting a victim think aloud without interruption, and the value of recreating the emotional aura of a crime scene in order to recapture suppressed detail. Questioning a suspect is different, however, and requires an aptitude to distinguish truth from lies. Sometimes it requires the wearing down of the perpetrator and even deception in order to gain a confession. Closed choices like: 'Did you mean to hurt Kevin with the gun or just scare him?' and even the articulation of the deliberate assumption of guilt are accepted ploys in criminal investigation. It is legally indefensible not to record a police interview for posterity whereas the doctor's clinical notes and letter to the general practitioner are the only permanent record of the confidential medical interview. Even if it is only what is said that ends up in the notes, paying attention to the way the patient gives the story is an essential element of getting people better.

I am immediately on my guard when a patient referred to see me for memory loss trails his wife into the consulting room and then informs me that there is nothing at all wrong and that he has no idea why he is here. When I ask him the day of the week or the month of the year and he turns backwards in the hope his wife will help him out, my suspicions of incipient dementia increase. The 'worried well', including those with anxious or obsessional personalities and people with dissociative states, often give very long-winded, overinclusive accounts of their forgetfulness or 'episodes of going blank' whereas people with early Alzheimer's disease give minimalist answers, look perplexed, or answer with face-saving humour. Some patients with cognitive impairment, especially those with frontotemporal dementia, confabulate to fill in memory gaps. Silent mouthing or exasperated facial gestures from the accompanying family often reinforce my suspicions that what I am hearing lacks credibility. People with depression may also be unable to remember. They often come over during the consultation as downcast, exhausted, inattentive and disengaged and answer questions with a laconic 'don't know'. I also see people who feign amnesia for some sort of gain such as the avoidance of criminal proceedings or a compensation claim after a road traffic accident. The medical history in these cases often takes over an hour to elicit and involves a great deal of collateral detective work including the perusal of medico-legal documents.

The information I gather during the medical interview is sometimes clear, but frequently shifting, often contradictory and inevitably incomplete. From time to time I encounter symptoms in the clinic that I have never heard before or that have yet to be acknowledged in the neurological literature. About five years ago a woman told me that for the last six months she had been bothered by an intermittent 'fizzy' feeling in the front of her left thigh which she likened to the feeling of a vibrating mobile phone. Two years ago a young marketing executive reported occasional flickering dots of static resembling a snowstorm in his field of vision and six weeks ago a university student told me that when he rubbed one of his eyes it made an audible squelching sound.

A vignette from my own casebook helps to illustrate the importance of listening in neurological diagnosis. Thirty-five years ago Mr Z, a forty-two-year-old plumber born in Gdansk, was referred to me at the now-closed Middlesex Hospital on Mortimer Street in London complaining of increasing stiffness and slowness. He had a stolid, staring facial expression and blinked very little. His posture was stooped and he dragged his legs when walking. When he sat down, two of the fingers of his left hand began to quiver. The referral letter from his general practitioner indicated that his symptoms had started ten weeks earlier. I went over the medical history with him, which gave me no clues as to the likely cause of his symptoms, but the physical examination confirmed my initial suspicion of Parkinson's syndrome. I organised a magnetic resonance head scan and started him on three daily capsules of L-DOPA, an amino acid precursor of the chemical messenger dopamine used to treat Parkinson's disease. I told him to double the dose after a week and asked him to come back to see me in eight weeks.

At his follow-up visit he strode in from the waiting room and informed me that he was cured. He looked ten years younger, had a smile on his face and his voice – which had been muffled and lacking in melody – was now loud and clear. I expressed my pleasure at this unexpected and spectacular transformation and informed him that his brain scan was normal. I then told him to stay on the L-DOPA tablets and come back to see me in a further three months. He then shook my hand and as an afterthought said that his girlfriend had asked him to enquire whether the Chinese herbs he had been taking for stress and high blood pressure might have been the cause. He then showed me a small white canister with a picture of plants and Mandarin writing inscribed on the front. Although I felt a causal relationship to be unlikely I asked him if he would mind waiting behind until I had seen the last patient of the morning. The two of us then walked down Cleveland Street to San Ling Chinese Medical Centre on Goodge Street where the herbalist told us that the treatment Mr Z was taking was called verticil and that the tablets contained extracts from a Rauwolfia species endemic in China. The snakeroot plant, as it is known in the West, contains an alkaloid called reserpine that depletes dopamine levels. After confirming that his girlfriend's suspicions were probably correct I advised Mr Z to stop taking the herbal medicine immediately and to tail his L-DOPA off over the next four weeks. At the final review he had fully recovered.

I knew that in the late nineteen-fifties reserpine had been used as an effective allopathic treatment for high blood pressure, but it had caused sedation and depression in many patients and Parkinson's syndrome in a few. Paying attention to a casual remark and following up in a way that some might today say was outside the line of duty had avoided Mr Z being labelled as having Parkinson's disease and receiving unneeded medication for the rest of his life.

Once I have completed the medical interview and the examination and ordered my thoughts I remind myself that patients are forced to remain silent while I am talking, either by choice, or as a consequence of the power I hold over them. I avoid assertive mono-logues, and deliberately leave gaps between sentences to allow them to absorb what I have said and space to respond. I try not to be the cause of fear by saying either too much or too little. Most people want a name for their distress, as it connects them to others with similar experiences and confirms that their symptoms fit within a recognised pattern. I never use big words when little ones are available, and I prefer for example to say 'loss of memory' than keep using the more hurt-ful word 'dementia'. How I give the diagnosis is one of the most important and challenging things I do as a doctor. I still remember how my heart sank when one of my chiefs at the National Hospital said with cold bluntness to a patient on the ward round, 'I know what you have, it is called motor neurone disease. I am afraid there is no cure and you have only about two years to live.'

Many of the diagnostic labels I confer on patients, such as cluster headaches and restless legs, were invented to offer coherence to poorly understood phenomena and to serve as a helpful shorthand to aid communication among healthcare professionals. More often than not, they give comfort rather than despair, but syndromes of dubious existence through the power of the word run the risk of creating an opaque shroud of ignorance that slows the recognition of more solid clinical entities.

When it comes to what can be done I explain the pros and cons of each option as impartially as possible. I paint the rosiest picture, based on the available evidence, and remind the patient that in modern medicine there are very few diseases that can be cured by a magic bullet. There are also situations where I need to mention that a medication can be highly effective for a distressing symptom even when the diagnosis is unknown. Every therapy in medicine has its disadvantages as well as benefits but I try to spend a greater amount of time emphasising what I know the recommended treatment can hope to achieve with anecdotes from my own experience. I encourage patients to express their own preferences and try to discuss openly their particular concerns about any of my recommendations. In order to help them come to a decision I sometimes say that almost everything in life, and most of what a doctor prescribes, is a trade-off. I do everything I can to optimise my placebo response and I keep in mind Kafka's country doctor's words to the family of a seriously ill man: 'To write prescriptions is easy but to come to an understanding with people is hard.' When I sense that the patient still has serious reservations about my advice I only force the issue of treatment if I feel there will be serious consequences in leaving things as they are.

Neurology has very few 'easy fixes' and the most powerful healer I have at my disposal is myself, not my prescription pad. Beaming into a patient's home can only ever be an inferior substitute for a face-to-face interview, giving any sort of bad news on a video consultation is inhumane, and attempts to carry out a neurological examination without touch is negligent. For straightforward minor patient queries, I have found the telephone to be a much better vehicle of communication with less sensory disconnection. Dr Stern told me that a doctor should always try to create a favourable impression but resist behaving like a salesman selling smart suits in a department store. I now understand how important the tone of my voice is in instilling confidence and in giving sympathy. I have also become better over time at dealing with patients' feelings of helplessness, hopelessness, denial and anger. Listening carefully is the single most effective method of making a neurological diagnosis and being heard is a transformative ritual that facilitates healing.

— The Dead Hospital —

Memories are random and volatile and defy logic. They are made in the dendritic canopy and appear and disappear as they wish. Some memories exist like delicately folded magic carpets; others lie covered in dust and forgotten in the kasbahs of the mind. Four years ago, I eventually succeeded in loosening the lid of a canister stored in my hippocampus which held a preserved engram of an undisturbed faraway time.

A red Routemaster left Camden Town and trundled around the Outer Circle, far enough away from the fence not to wake the sleeping animals. The next sequence showed me alighting from the bus at St John's Wood with a security guard and a cleaner. I then crossed Park Road and hugged the high perimeter wall of the cricket ground as far as the Grace Gates. When I reached the grand mansions of Hamilton Terrace I seemed to be scuffing my right foot. On arriving at Maida Vale I sat watching a cavalcade of hussars heading for their barracks on Albany Street. In the bushes behind the bench the familiar flute of a male blackbird reassured me I was in time.

Two gables bookended the hospital's brick façade, and its upper-floor balconies had iron balustrades supported by a rig of unsightly scaffolding. An out-of-town ambulance with its back door thrown open was parked in the vacant forecourt. A little to the right of the chimney stack, a small brick outhouse with a wooden door marked the spot where wartime bombing had blown up the roof. An arch had been cut through the southerly gable leading to the back of the hospital and the medical school.

As the noise of rolling tyres and the braking and acceleration of vehicles began to get louder and drown out the birdsong I walked up the curved stone steps buttressed by pairs of Corinthian columns, through a glass-panelled door and into a narrow corridor that ran parallel to the front of the hospital. I climbed the flight of stairs that led up to the wards. The cathedral-like silence of the hospital was broken only by the lift cage slamming shut, followed by the echoing rumble of its ascent to the operating theatre. I was wearing a white coat and a silk guards tie, and my black leather shoes shone brightly thanks to the daily application before leaving home of Cherry Blossom polish. I looked youthful and intense as I sat in Sister Margaret Mary Lynch's office writing up my notes.

These greyscale motion pictures stored in buried spools return now whenever I cast my mind back once more to Maida Vale. I have similar reels for the other lost hospitals where I trained, Mile End Hospital on Bancroft Road, Poplar on the East India Dock Road, St Stephen's on the Fulham Road, New End, the Cruciform building on Gower Street, The Middlesex Hospital and Pavilion 12A of the Highlands Hospital on Worlds End Lane. All of them have laid dormant in their cans uncorrupted by the lies of constant remembering, forgetting and re-remembering.

Maida Vale Hospital for Nervous Diseases was the culmination of an idea conceived originally by a German-born physician and polymath called Julius Althaus, who had studied nervous diseases with Charcot in Paris and, after emigrating to England, had worked as an assistant to Robert Bentley Todd at King's College Hospital where he had further developed his interest in electrotherapy. Todd had a special interest

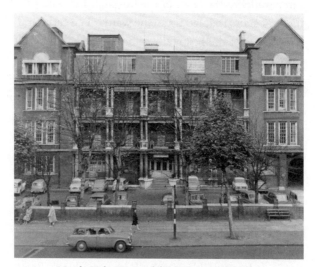

Maida Vale Hospital for Nervous Diseases,
4 Maida Vale, London W9 (1963).

in physiological medicine and had already written a well-received textbook on diseases of the brain and other afflictions of the nervous system before Althaus started to train with him. He is now best known by neurologists for his description of temporary focal paralysis that follows an epileptic convulsion and which he ascribed to exhaustion of the motor cortex.

Althaus believed there was a need for another specialist hospital for nervous diseases in addition to the National Hospital for the Paralysed and Epileptic in Queen Square, opened in 1860, and the London Galvanic Hospital, established by Dr Harry Lobb in Cavendish Square a year later, and raised funds to create The London Infirmary for Epilepsy and Paralysis in a house on Charles Street, now Blandford Place. The Brahmin physicians at the large London teaching hospitals disapproved of these boutique hospitals that were sprouting up all over London at that time and accused their founders of self-interest masquerading as philanthropy or scientific advance. Their proliferation led to a caustic editorial that appeared in the *Lancet* in 1863:

These excrescences are being reproduced with all the prolific exuberance characteristic of malignancy and soon the metropolis threatens to swarm with nuisances of this kind . . . next may come a Quinine Hospital, a hospital for Treatment by Cod-Liver Oil by the Hypophosphites or by the Excrement of Boa Constrictors.

Despite this snub from the medical establishment, Althaus's tiny hospital survived and soon gained a reputation for its application of electrical stimulation to alleviate chronic nervous disorders. When the five-year lease expired in Charles Street in 1872, the hospital moved to larger premises at Winterton House in Portland Terrace, on the north side of Regent's Park, where it became known as The Hospital for Epilepsy and Paralysis. It was there on 25 November 1884 that the first successful extirpation of a brain tumour in the world occurred. The patient, a twenty-five-year-old Scottish farmer named Henderson, had been admitted into one of the hospital's twenty beds because of severe weakness in his left arm and a milder loss of strength in his left leg. Over the preceding three years he had also experienced frequent seizures, which affected the left side of his face and his tongue and caused his head to turn involuntarily to the left side. The physician in charge of his case, Dr Alexander Hughes Bennett, had taken advantage of research carried out by David Ferrier, a former member of staff at the hospital, to localise the site of mischief to the upper part of the fissure of Rolando in the right cerebral hemisphere. His findings on examination had included swollen optic discs indicative of raised pressure in the brain, a left hemiparesis that was most severe in the arm and pathologically brisk tendon reflexes on the left side.

Ferrier, who was born and educated in Aberdeen and had studied logic, philosophy and psychology before taking up medical studies at the University of Edinburgh, is now regarded as one of the giants of British neurology. His first medical post was as an assistant to a general practitioner in Bury St Edmunds where he spent much of his spare time carrying out studies in comparative anatomy in his sponsor's large garden. His most important work was carried out in the animal research laboratory of the West Riding Pauper Lunatic Asylum before he moved to London, where he was able to confirm using faradic electrical stimulation the cerebral organisation of coordinated movement and localise the areas in the monkey brain responsible for arm retraction, walking, tongue protrusion and wrist extension. Bennett's father had died of a potentially operable brain tumour and it was this that motivated him to pressurise a thirty-five-year-old surgeon called Rickman Godlee to try to relieve Henderson's suffering. The day after the operation, *The Times* reported that several of London's most eminent physicians, including the father of British neurology, John Hughlings Jackson, had been present in the hospital's operating theatre to watch Godlee make a one-inch trephine opening in the skull and remove a transparent lobulated tumour that was about the size of a walnut. Half an hour after the operation Henderson was able to answer questions coherently but on the fourth postoperative day the wound became infected leading to his death a month later. This landmark event in the history of brain surgery enhanced the hospital's reputation and contributed to it fulfilling Althaus's dream of becoming a serious competitor to the National Hospital for the Paralysed and Epileptic in Queen Square.

Althaus's brainchild continued to flourish after his death in 1900 and, as a result of renewed medical entrepreneurship, the hospital moved again in 1903, this time to 4 Maida Vale, where its unprepossessing appearance belied the high standards of medicine that were practised in its operating theatres and wards. In 1937 its name changed yet again to Maida Vale Hospital for Nervous Diseases (including Epilepsy and Paralysis) by which time it was pioneering the use of phenobarbitone in the treatment of fits and was at the forefront of a new technique to record brain wave rhythms as an aid to the diagnosis of epilepsy. One of the hospital's most renowned physicians and teachers between the wars was Lord Russell Brain and his presence on the staff attracted young neurologists and neurosurgeons from all over the world. Almost all of the eighty-two beds in the hospital were taken up by complex and esoteric neurological disorders that had been referred for diagnosis and treatment from every part of the United Kingdom, and even though there was no acute emergency department, Maida Vale Hospital for Nervous Diseases was the polar opposite of a cottage hospital, or a home for the incurable.

When I began to work there as a registrar in 1979, Maida Vale – as we called it – had already been amalgamated with its old rival, the National Hospital in

Queen Square, for over thirty years, but had managed to preserve a distinctive identity. Unlike another diminutive specialist hospital called the West End Hospital for Nervous Diseases at 91 Dean Street, Soho, which had been viewed by many of the senior physicians at Queen Square up to its closure in 1972 as a second-rate place, Maida Vale was considered a proper – if marginally inferior – hospital. There was still a great sense of camaraderie and a continuity of tradition that had disappeared in some of London's premier teaching hospitals as a result of their physical dislocation into new impersonal flagship skyscrapers. As you came in from the main entrance of the hospital into the waiting room of the bijou outpatient department there were twenty comfortable chairs neatly arranged around tables and against one wall a worn-out piano that was still regularly used by the staff after hours. Louise, the nursing sister, and Clover, her assistant, served tea and coffee on trays to the patients who sat sedately, some leafing through copies of *The Lady* or *Country Life*. In my mind's eye I can see myself sitting behind a desk in one of the four consulting rooms talking to a woman with a beehive and a foot drop. I am laughing heartily as she tells me how her Labrador dog had begun to imitate her limp when she took it for walks in Little Venice.

On Tuesdays, once clinic was over, I used to go down the small wooden staircase that led to the microscope room. Robin Osler Barnard, my teacher, arrived on the dot of nine o'clock every morning dressed in a bowler hat and smart navy-blue overcoat, carrying a small leather briefcase. He had an elfin face, a comb-over hairstyle and wore thick glasses with round frames. Most of the year he was dressed in a three-piece suit and wore wing-collar shirts with a bow tie or cravat, but in the summer months he would arrive sporting a boater and a blue blazer and carrying a large umbrella. He was a quaint traveller from an antique land determined to preserve falling standards, but what he taught me about pathology was of immense contemporary value. Barnard worked alone and had a gentlemanly approach to his métier. His tutorials always began with his secretary offering us a cup of Earl Grey tea and a slice of Dundee cake. He would show us photographs of brains, read extracts from the actual case notes and get his assistant to project lantern slides showing images of diseased brain tissue.

One day he pulled out a preserved brain section about three centimetres thick and while holding it up told us that it had belonged to a Lieutenant Colonel in the Indian army. The officer had started to have severe morning headaches and vomiting and had died a few weeks later as a result of a bout of grand mal seizures that had lasted several hours. He went on to say that when he had examined the brain with the naked eye he had noted that it was strafed with wormholes caused by the inadvertent ingestion of the eggs of a pork tapeworm. He then pulled out a Mason jar containing a single diaphanous vesicle floating in formaldehyde and said that it was much more common to find a solitary large larval cyst in the brain than the many small ones that had killed the soldier. He then pointed out that attached to the cyst's inner membrane was a small nodule that contained a double row of hooks and four cushion-shaped suckers. This single giant one-centimetre hydatid had been successfully removed from the brain of a Bengali restaurant owner in a heroic operation carried out by Mr Wylie McKissock in the Maida Vale operating theatre. We then waited in line to see what he had marked for us to focus on in the sections of the Indian officer's brain. His own observations were frequently framed as Socratic questions such as 'I wonder what that is?' and I never recall him telling me that I'd misidentified something. Through his benevolence I was learning by example to make the most of a light microscope.

Under Barnard's tutelage I learned to distinguish neurones from glial stars, identify the nucleus of a cell, and recognise abnormal mitotic figures. He also introduced me to the line and colour of cerebral tissue and the world of the infinitely small. I learned the value of the colourful chemistry of dyes that William Morris had used in his fabric workshop at 26 Queen Square. On one occasion he showed me a crimson nucleus surrounded by yellow cytoplasm on a green background that had been stained with anilines. This rainbow of tints allowed him to reveal the extent of a patient's disease and its intricate complexity. With a wry grin he told me that the number of neurones in the brain was the same as the number of stars in the Milky Way, so extrapolation was an accepted method of cell counting. He would say to us that a neurologist with no appreciation of pathology was the equivalent of an apprentice car mechanic who had never opened the bonnet of a car to look at the engine.

His way of speaking left me spellbound. I learned later that it was the particular diction of a man who had trained at St Thomas' Hospital. In those days it was possible to have a reasonable stab at the name of the London teaching hospital where a colleague had trained by certain expressions they used and their particular way of pronouncing words.

He also had impeccable manners and it was a great shock when I noticed that he had dirty fingernails. I was also amused that he always ate his sandwiches prepared at home on the same table where he conducted the brain cuts. Along the corridor from his office was a room that housed a state-of-the-art electron microscope where Michael Kidd had first identified the paired helical filament that characterised the ultramicroscopic appearance of Alzheimer's disease in 1963. We never went in, and I formed the impression that he considered it a complex piece of unnecessary kit that had little impact on his own ability to diagnose 'monstrocellular sarcomas'.

In another of his seminars he taught me that in 1873 the 'black reaction' discovered by the Italian biologist and pathologist Camillo Golgi had been a critical step in the visualisation of nerve cells and the surrounding connective tissue. Santiago Ramón y Cajal had then used this new technique to silver the cerebrum and demonstrate irrefutably that each neurone was an autonomous unit that made contact with its neighbours through protoplasmic kisses (now known as synapses). Cajal likened the pyramidal cells of the cortex to trees which, if nurtured, could grow fresh branches and roots.

The morgue, tucked away in an unvisited part of the hospital, was the lair of Dougal, a pasty-faced man with an oblong-shaped head and a sonorous voice. He told me that he had lost his ability to smell human remains. When I got to know him better I realised he had a complete indifference to life and a loathing of humanity. Once, as we were eating our fish and chips together in the hospital canteen, he told me that he believed the soul remained in the brain after it had been removed from the cadaver and that even when it had been fixed in formalin, a brain never lost its mind. To lighten the mood I teased him that there were not many bodies coming in at the moment and that he might need to do something about it. He then put his hand over his mouth and whispered that he had a corpse bagged up in the freezer and that Dr Barnard would be performing the autopsy later that afternoon.

Dr Barnard and Dougal were already dressed in surgical attire when I arrived at the mortuary and were bent over an emaciated cadaver that lay supine on a stainless-steel table. Dougal had written the height and weight of the corpse down on a whiteboard. Barnard then began the post-mortem examination by confirming aloud the name of the deceased as written on his armband. He then turned in my direction and said that the man had died in another hospital of what was thought to have been a stroke, but he had been treated for many years before that at Maida Vale for a mysterious and ill-defined frontal lobe degeneration. The family and patient had consented to a diagnostic post-mortem examination before death and the body had been transferred to Maida Vale in an ambulance.

Barnard then made a long Y-shaped incision from the neck down to the pubic bone with a PM 40 knife while at the same time mentioning that the cause of death written by the physician on the certificate was wrong, or only partially correct in two of every three post-mortem examinations he performed. After cutting through muscle and opening the abdominal wall he then palpated the liver, spleen, pancreas and stomach. A soup ladle was used to collect fluid from the peritoneal cavity before he severed the thirty feet of guts just below the pylorus and at the lower rectum, and then unravelled and removed intestines from the body like a long string of dripping sausages. Next he cut through the ribs and removed the breastbone with a pair of shears, releasing the lungs with a cradling motion. Once he had carefully removed each lung from the thoracic cavity he squeezed them, looking for oedema, before proceeding to remove the heart. Once the heart was in his hands he rinsed it with water before inserting his fingers into its valves. Each precious organ was then placed on a tray, and weighed and carefully examined for signs of disease.

Meanwhile Dougal had made a single incision just below the ears, across the back of the head, and had carefully peeled back the scalp and the muscles from the skull with the front skin flap resting over the face and the back flap hanging loosely over the nape. He had then used a rotating saw to create a bony skull-cap which he had lifted up with a chisel to expose the brain. With the aid of a scalpel he then extricated the brain from the cranial cavity with his fingers leaving the spinal cord in place. Barnard scrutinised the brain for several minutes and told me he could see no bleeds, focal areas of softening or any hardening of the linings. The brain was then wrapped in formalin-soaked towels in preparation for fixation and subsequent careful examination under the microscope. The autopsy was almost complete, and it was Dougal's job to make the cadaver presentable again, which he did with the help of twine, glue, cotton wool and sticking plaster. He then washed and groomed the deceased. I had spent an afternoon immersing myself in what is regarded in medicine as the ultimate audit and I remember afterwards feeling especially vibrant and alive.

By the time I had joined the consultant staff at

Maida Vale in 1983, after working there for the previous two years as a senior registrar, the mortuary had been closed down because of health and safety concerns. Dougal had been made redundant and rumours circulated that he was working as an extra in some of the last of the Hammer horror films. The long-promised building maintenance was never carried out and, to make matters worse, management started to employ more agency staff, which coincided directly with a palpable diminution in the communal sense of purpose. The hospital I loved had started to resemble a dying coral reef. Sometimes I would go to see Barnard in his office to seek solace. He never seemed to mind my interruptions and his calm presence reassured me that all was well with the world. I now knew that his dirty fingernails could be explained by his passion for vintage cars of which he had a small collection at his country home. Tamas Revesz, his senior registrar, had also told me that he was regularly invited to judge at the Pebble Beach Concours d'Elegance in California.

As in the former times of my training Barnard would order some tea, pull out the boxes of slides and then say, 'Let's look at it.' There was one occasion when we studied an archival case of subacute spongiform encephalopathy, one of a series of eight cases published by his predecessor W. H. McMenemey along with his neurologist colleague, Sam Nevin. Three of these patients had been operated on in the theatre of the hospital between one and two years before developing the deadly disease and Barnard suspected that there had been transmission from surgical instruments of an as-yet unidentified infectious agent. He then pulled out the battered visitors' book and showed me the autographs of Ludo van Bogaert from Antwerp, Walter R. Kirschbaum from Chicago, Serge Brion from Paris and the Nobel Laureate Carleton Gajdusek, all of whom had made pilgrimages to Maida Vale and delivered lectures at the hospital on kuru and Creutzfeldt-Jakob disease.

Another episode of the film comes back clearly now as I resume writing. I am on call for the night and as the first bats start to fly over the outhouses on St John's Wood Road, I leave the doctor's residence and clatter down the perilous open steel stairwell to walk the short distance to the medical school building. The patients who had attended for physiotherapy earlier in the day had all left and the wooden door on the ground floor is locked. I climb up the stairs and open the anatomical museum with the key I had signed for earlier that day. In the middle of the room is a large rectangular wooden table surrounded on all sides by shelves of specimens. These brains, whether embedded in blocks or floating free, continued to have a presence and purpose even after death. I pick up a pot with a faded label that contains a swollen brain with flattened convolutions. Its hind brain has been compressed by an expanding fibrous neoplasm, which has infiltrated the left hemisphere and forced the midline structures over to the opposite side completely obliterating the left lateral ventricle. The tumour is solid in some parts and cystic in others and within its substance I can make out areas of necrosis and bleeding. I then turn my attention to the spinal cord suspended with the help of fine cotton strings in a large glass jar filled with sepia-tinted liquid. A serpentine proliferation of veins and capillaries on its surface had caused the vertebral bone to erode.

There were nights on call when I dreamt of my own brain, encased in the penumbra of a faceless head inside the serrated seams of a white skull. I never dared to touch it, but I watched fascinated as it throbbed and wept. Maida Vale was a time when I was very much caught up with my own pathology.

Time and change finally brought down the curtain on the hospital that I loved and had worked at for fifteen years. The Holy House, with its medical school of impressionistic art, was boarded up, symbolising the death of innocence. The hospital remained desolate for two more years, guarded by savage dogs, until in the last days of the summer of 1995 bulldozers and wrecking balls arrived and razed it to the ground. Its demise was more than the end of an era. The changes that were happening in the National Health Service were now forcing me to become a smiling handshaker who got on well with people, especially managers and governors. The only consolation was that I still had a job that I enjoyed.

— Zadig and Voltaire —

J oseph Bell, the Edinburgh surgeon whose clinical methods Arthur Conan Doyle later claimed were the blueprint for his fictional character Sherlock Holmes, revealed the source of his own diagnostic approach in a short review published in the December 1892 edition of *The Bookman*:

There is nothing new under the sun: Voltaire taught us the method of Zadig, and every good teacher of medicine or surgery exemplifies every day in his teaching and practice the method and its results. The precise and intelligent recognition and appreciation of minor differences is the real essential factor in all successful medical diagnosis.

Bell's reference compels us to go back to Voltaire's wonderful fable, *The Book of Fate*, published in 1747, where, weary of the iniquities of Babylon, Zadig the philosopher hero flees to the banks of the Euphrates to study nature in all its godly detail. When the chief eunuch of the Queen comes by looking for a stray dog, Zadig asks him whether the missing animal is a small bitch with puppies and a lame left leg. In great excitement the eunuch demands to know where the dog is, only for Zadig to reply that he has never set eyes on it but that tracks in the sand, disturbed pebbles and some recently snapped twigs had allowed him to construct a picture of the animal in his mind. Voltaire's description of Zadig's skill in abductive reasoning was itself derivative, being based on a translation of a sixteenth-century collection of stories about the travels of the three sons of the King of Serendippo.

Bell was aware of the importance of the infinitely minuscule that allowed him to make distinctions where others saw only monotonous uniformity. One day a woman accompanied by a small child was brought to his clinic at the Royal Infirmary. He exchanged greetings and, while observing her with his sharp piercing grey eyes, casually asked:

'What sort o' crossing did ye have from Burntisland?'
'It was good,' she answered.
'And had ye a good walk up Inverleith Row?'
'Yes.'
'And what did ye do with the other wain?'
'I left him with my sister in Leith.'
'And would ye still be working at the linoleum factory?'
'Yes, I am.'

He explained to his students that the woman before them had a distinguishing Fife accent that he had been able to place as soon as she spoke. When she sat down he had noticed an inflamed blistered rash on her fingers, an occupational dermatitis caused by pine rosin that he knew was used in the linoleum factory in Burntisland. He then pointed out the red clay on the sides of her shoes which, in Edinburgh, was only found in the Botanical Gardens. The most direct route from Leith to the hospital would have taken the woman down Inverleith Row, which bordered the gardens. Lastly, he had observed that the coat she was carrying over her arm was too large for the little child, and so he had assumed she must have an older boy.

Bell considered that it was Conan Doyle's own medical training which had provided him with the model for his famous detective's modus operandi:

Conan Doyle's education as a student of medicine taught him how to observe, and his practice, both as a general practitioner and a specialist, has been a splendid training for a man such as he is, gifted with eyes, memory, and imagination. Eyes and ears which can see and hear, memory to record at once and to recall at pleasure the impressions of the senses, and an imagination capable of weaving a theory or piecing together a broken chain, or unravelling a tangled clue, such are implements of his trade to a successful diagnostician.

Included within the sixty Sherlock Holmes adventures are references to sixty-eight diseases, thirty-two medical terms, thirty-eight doctors, twenty-two drugs, twelve medical specialties, six hospitals and even three medical journals and two medical schools.

Another of Doyle's influences may have been the work of Giovanni Morelli, an art historian who had studied medicine in Switzerland and Germany and taught anatomy at the University of Munich. Morelli wrote that the aesthetic beauty of the human ear depended on its oval shell-like shape bounded on the outside by a well-defined helix and at the bottom by a developed lobule. By paying attention to discrepancies in the portrayal of the human ear Morelli had acquired a connoisseurship that allowed him to detect art fakes purporting to be the work of the Grand Masters.

In an influential essay on conjectural science entitled 'On the Method of Zadig', published in 1881, T. H. Huxley concluded that:

For the rigorous application of Zadig's logic to the results of accurate and long-continued observation has founded all those sciences that have been termed historical or palaetiological, because they are retrospectively prophetic and strive towards the reconstruction in human imagination of events that have vanished and ceased to be.

In Arthur Conan Doyle's Sherlock Holmes stories, Dr Watson is intrigued by the eccentric behaviour and single-mindedness of his new flatmate who tells him that whether the earth rotates round the sun or vice versa is of no concern or interest to him. He discovers that Holmes has a sound background in chemistry and is an expert in trivia such as cigarette ash, plant poisons and shirtsleeves, but is ignorant of literature, politics and philosophy. In the process of trying to discern Holmes' profession Watson remarks: 'No man burdens his mind with small matters unless he has some very good reason for doing so.'

In *The Hound of the Baskervilles* Holmes explains to his friend that in order to avoid his brain becoming over-cluttered, he retains only those facts which may help him solve future criminal investigations:

Students of criminology will remember the analogous incidents in Grodno, in Little Russia, in the year '66, and of course there are the Anderson murders in North Carolina, but this case possesses some features which are entirely its own.

I found it easy to engage with the character of Sherlock Holmes as he reminded me of some of my teachers. Watson observed: 'You're like a surgeon who wants every symptom before he can give a diagnosis.' 'Exactly,' Holmes responded. 'That expresses it. And it is only a patient who has an object in deceiving his surgeon who would conceal the facts of his case.' Holmes was the superhero of material reason, half-doctor, half-virtuoso, who used his luminous intellect to solve insoluble problems. After being shown a single fact in all its bearings he was able to deduce the chain of events that led up to the crime and the consequences that followed. On his very first case he tells Watson:

I have already explained to you that what is out of the common is usually a guide rather than a hindrance. In solving a problem of this sort, the grand thing is to be able to reason backwards. That is a very useful accomplishment, and a very easy one, but people do not practise it much. In the everyday affairs of life it is more useful to reason forwards, and so the other comes to be neglected. There are fifty who can reason synthetically for one who can reason analytically.

The unreal universe of Sherlock Holmes was my primer in neurology and it soon became a bridge to Dr William Gowers, arguably the greatest neurologist that ever lived. In his 1905 clinical lecture 'A Metastatic Mystery', transcribed verbatim by his assistants using phonographic shorthand and then published in the *Lancet*, Gowers described aspects of his method that bore an uncanny similarity with those used by the Baker Street sleuth:

When I say you cannot have too much of diagnostic method I mean that the power you will hereafter need, the power of discerning the nature of disease, can only be gained by constant exercise. You should systematically follow the process of diagnosis in every case observing its elements and their relative weight. Avoid the easy habit of taking in the diagnosis as a whole and being satisfied with the recognition of the disease. It is only by thoughtful perception of the reasoning, which varies in detail in every case that you can gain the ability to deal in like manner with cases that are unfamiliar. The power will come unconsciously.

Gowers searched for commonalities and exceptions that would allow him to disclose where, and why, a particular part of the nervous system was faulty. Both neurologists and criminal detectives seek hidden truths and meanings in complicated and often contradictory data. They also rely on a rigorous tried-and-tested method which pays attention to detail: identification of clues hinges on the skills of inquiry and inspection and without them there is unlikely to be a successful outcome.

When I arrived at the National Hospital in Queen Square in 1979 to continue my training, it was an experience akin to entering the Valley of the Kings at Luxor. I was surrounded everywhere by the ghosts of distinguished physicians like Brown-Séquard, Ferrier and Jackson, and it felt as if some were still haunting the wards. There were instances when I could feel Gowers' penetrating blue eyes watching me at the bedside and hear his harsh staccato voice reminding me that neurology was a personal science that depended on exactness of observation and constant reasoning from the facts:

Discard in the first instance all attempts to identify or to name, and try instead to read the malady, tracing the symptoms to the seat of their cause, and discerning the nature of the morbid process by their character and course.

Queen Square had been laid out in 1716 with fashionable Georgian terraces on three sides, leaving the north side open so its wealthy residents could admire the picturesque views of Hampstead Heath. In the middle of the nineteenth century a seismic transformation occurred with a procession of institutions devoted to health, education and other charitable works replacing many of the private houses. Since then it has changed relatively little and it is still a desirable and peaceful Bloomsbury hideaway that can only be accessed by ambulance through two narrow streets. The Queen's Larder tavern, the church of St George the Martyr and the statue of Queen Charlotte at the north end of the lawn are three of its best-known historical landmarks. There were two other surviving hospitals from the nineteenth century: one was the white stucco Ospedale Italiano, a private institution with just forty-eight beds and a small clinic run by an excellent Italian general practitioner who took care of the surviving Italian community of Clerkenwell. The neurosurgeons from the National Hospital sometimes admitted private patients there and it was a privilege to go and clerk them in before their operations. Sisters of St Vincent de Paul with their distinctive uniforms still provided some of the care. The other medical institution was the Royal Homeopathic Hospital, which was in decline despite its royal patronage. Just round the corner in Great Ormond Street was the world-famous Children's Hospital.

The National Hospital for Nervous Diseases, now called the National Hospital for Neurology and

Neurosurgery, had a gabled roof and small regimented windows. Most passers-by did not even realise it was a hospital. The chief porter would sometimes stand at the entrance as smartly dressed as the commissionaire outside Claridge's hotel. Inside, figures in striped pyjamas with half-moon scars visible on their shaved heads limped and shuffled down the labyrinthine corridors. In outpatients, a cortex of neurologists were busy hunting for diagnostic clues that would provide answers and solve problems. Next to the Old Board Room and to the right of the front entrance was the chapel, and further down the main corridor on the left was the Gowers Library with its highbrow selection of newspapers and periodicals. My first impressions were more of a rather shabby gentleman's club than an august cradle of healing.

Not long after I had started my post as junior registrar on the 'Marshall firm', I was involved in a real-life crime case. I was called by Iris, the sister on the Batten Intensive Care Unit, to see a chartered accountant who had been transferred from another hospital with loss of power in his legs. The man told me that he had become ill a week earlier with vomiting, abdominal pain and diarrhoea which had resolved without treatment but just as he had started to feel better he had developed severe burning pain in his legs. The doctor who had examined him in the Accident and Emergency Department noted foot drop due to reduced power and admitted him to hospital. Over the next two days he became weaker and the pain worsened leading to his ultimate transfer to Queen Square. He now had reduced strength in all the muscles of his legs, but more so in his feet, and his tendon reflexes were absent. Analysis of his spinal fluid revealed an elevated protein, a normal glucose level and no white cells, findings that supported the diagnosis of Guillain-Barré syndrome, an immunological disorder of the peripheral nerves. After his admission he continued to deteriorate, he was hardly able to move his legs at all and the weakness ascended to involve his arms, respiratory muscles and face. One of the nurses reported that his hair was falling out. He remained paralysed and delirious on a ventilator for the next two weeks. At this point the institutional memory of the hospital came to the rescue when one of the other consultants on the staff was invited to give an opinion and recalled that he had seen a similar case. Shortly after he had started working at Queen Square, a warehouseman at a photographic supplies company near St Albans had been transferred with severe paralysis of the arms and legs and weakness of his facial muscles and eyelids. The illness had started with what was thought to be gastric flu and had been followed by painful pins and needles in the soles of the feet. He also remembered that the man had developed an excoriated scaly rash on his face and scrotum before dying in agony a few days after admission. Iris then nodded that she too recalled the man. At the time fifty-six-year-old Fred Biggs had

gone down in criminal history as the second victim of
Graham Young, 'The Teacup Poisoner' who, during
his long subsequent confinement in Broadmoor, pre-
ferred the nickname, 'The World Poisoner'. On post-
mortem examination, large amounts of thallium had
been found in Mr Biggs's brain and peripheral nerves.

Our patient's urine and blood were checked for
thallium but came back negative, so the diagnosis of
Guillain-Barré remained unchanged. About a week
later I noticed for the first time some white bands of
discolouration on the patients nails that a dermatolo-
gist who walked across from University College Hospital confirmed were Mees' Lines, a sign of heavy metal
toxicity. Thallium poisoning was again back on the
differential diagnosis and with the help of the Metropolitan Police Toxicology Laboratory we were able
to detect raised levels of thallium in a sample of the
man's pubic hair. For the first and last time in my
career I wrote a prescription for Prussian blue, a syn-
thetic pigment, prepared as a colloidal dispersion by
the oxidation of ferrous ferrocyanide salts, and which
has the potential to chelate thallium. The man slowly
recovered and was discharged. A *crime passionnel* was
suspected but never proved.

I learned from Critchley's biography that William
Gowers had been a reserved man with few close friends
and there had been unsubstantiated rumours that he
had become dependent on opium and Indian hemp

after developing severe sciatica. During his formative years working as an apprentice to the apothecary
Thomas Simpson in Coggeshall in 1862, he had begun
to make meticulous observations on the wildflowers of
Essex. This botanical study was part of the mandatory
preparation for the University of London matricula-
tion examination and taught him to observe without
prejudice and record precisely what he had seen. It was
during these formative years that he began his lifelong
hobby of etching and engraving and doing pencil
drawings of plants and watercolour paintings of land-
scapes. In his inaugural address delivered at the opening of the First Session of Instruction at the National
Hospital, Queen Square, and published in the October
1896 issue of the *Lancet*, he told his audience:

The difference between adequate and inadequate observation,
between precision and laxity, between looking and seeing is
more than a difference in degree; it is absolute, and absolute
also is the enduring influence.

By reading his lectures during my training I came
to realise that in medical diagnosis there was never
absolute perfection, never an opinion that was beyond
rebuttal, and that one must always consider possible
alternatives, and provide against them. Rather than
try to frame a collection of baffling symptoms into
a diagnostic label that would stick and then be hard
to remove it was better to accept ignorance. He also

warned that a doctor's thinking could easily become anchored to specific reference points and so run the risk of error:

Our thought is apt to run in grooves from which it does not readily escape . . . and I would urge you to cultivate the habit of viewing a chronic case afresh from time to time; ignore what you have thought of it; put yourself in the face of a fresh observer and try and see if it thus bears a new aspect.

Another point Gowers often made when teaching his class was that if everything else pointed to a particular diagnosis then the absence of a single pathognomonic sign should never rule it out. This sort of inclusive error is sometimes referred to in medicine as the crime of Procrustes – the inclination to fit the facts to our opinions instead of our opinions to the facts. Procrustes was a figure in Greek mythology who offered unwitting travellers a bed for the night. Little did they know that he would then amputate their legs or stretch them to fit his one-size-fits-all bed.

Certain symptoms are very frequent in a given disease. Their presence may make that disease certain; but their absence does not prove that the disease does not exist. Neglect of this rule is a frequent source of error.

Inspector Gregory says to Holmes in 'The Adventure of Silver Blaze':

'Is there any other point to which you would wish to draw my attention?'
'To the curious incident of the dog in the night-time.'
'The dog did nothing in the night-time.'
'That was the curious incident,' remarked Sherlock Holmes.

Fictional characters often have origins in the life-time experiences of their creators. There was an intellectual depth to Sherlock Holmes that suggested there might be some additional precursor in addition to Bell and Morelli. Conan Doyle was interested in neurology and knew about recent scientific advances in the speciality from his research on vasomotor changes in tabes dorsalis, which he submitted as a thesis for the degree of Doctor of Medicine several years after graduating from Edinburgh University. I started to convince myself that he must have read Gowers' account in the *Manual of Diseases of the Nervous System* for his description of the Russian nobleman's feigned catalepsy in 'The Adventure of the Resident Patient'. Then, in a flight of fancy, I also imagined Doyle walking on the opposite side of Queen Square to visit the London Spiritualist Alliance while Gowers was teaching in the hospital. I then dreamt up a meeting of Gowers and Doyle in the home of Rudyard Kipling.

One of my favourite Sherlock Holmes tales is 'The Adventure of the Cardboard Box', first published in *The Strand* magazine of January 1893. Holmes reads in the paper that a Miss Susan Cushing, a fifty-year-old spinster of Cross Street, Croydon, has received a parcel in the post that contains two severed ears packed in salt. Holmes and Watson travel down to Croydon to meet with Inspector Lestrade who suspects it to be a prank carried out by three medical students that Miss Cushing had been forced to evict because of unruly behaviour, basing his suspicion in part on the fact that the parcel had been posted from Belfast, the hometown of one of the students. After noticing that a tarred string often used by sailors had been used to secure the contents of the box and that the address on its front revealed a spelling correction Holmes is convinced that a serious crime has been committed. The crude severance of the two pierced ears, one sun-burned and discoloured from a male and the other small and finely formed from a female, plus the use of salt as a preservative, implicates an unschooled person with links to the sea and who is not familiar with Croydon. He next inspects each ear carefully and notices that the smaller and more delicate of them possessed the same broad curve of the upper lobe, the short pinna and convolution of the inner cartilage as Miss Cushing's own ear. After a few further inquiries relating to Miss Cushing's two sisters and a visit to one of them Holmes hands Lestrade one of his visiting cards with the name of the murderer written on the back.

That evening over cigars at 221B Baker Street Holmes tells Watson that as in *A Study in Scarlet* and

The Sign of the Four it had been necessary to reason backwards from effects to causes. He reminds Watson that as a medical man he must be aware that there is no part of human anatomy as varied as the ear and that each ear is distinctive and differs from all other ones. He then tells him that he had recently written two essays on the topic in the *Anthropological Journal* and was therefore able to examine the evidence as an expert. Holmes' investigations lead to the prompt arrest of a ship's steward called Jim Browner for the double murder of his wife Mary, Susan Cushing's sister, and her lover Alec Fairbairn.

Apart from palpating the pinna for uric acid tophi in suspected gout and looking in the external auditory meatus for the blisters of shingles in people presenting to the emergency department with Bell's palsy, I had paid very little attention to the human ear until Karen Doherty, one of my research fellows, commented on the low-set ears of a young man who had been diagnosed with Parkinson's disease. After the ward round was finished we refreshed our knowledge of the anatomical parts of the external ear, and then consulted an online atlas of human malformations that had been associated with particular chromosomal abnormalities and birth defects. The closest match was DiGeorge syndrome, a rare hereditary disease caused by a microdeletion in the 22q11 chromosome. The ears in this condition are described as cupped with a thick overfolded helix and deep auricular pits. We went back to the ward and by knowing what to look for we were able to confirm that the patient also had slightly hooded eyes and a broad bridge of the nose, other recognised features of DiGeorge syndrome. A week later the results of the chromosomal analysis confirmed the diagnosis.

DiGeorge syndrome usually manifests itself in childhood with epileptic fits due to low calcium levels, floppy limbs, congenital anomalies of the heart, kidney and palate and a predisposition to recurrent infections. In adolescence it can present with acute anxiety or symptoms resembling schizophrenia but in 2013 there were only a handful of reports linking it to Parkinson's syndrome. This casual bedside observation would later lead to a genetic research project which showed that there was a fifty-fold increased risk of Parkinson's disease in DiGeorge syndrome and that one in 200 patients presenting with Parkinsonism before the age of forty possessed this particular chromosome deletion.

After Karen's diagnostic coup I paid much more attention to the appearance of ears. A deep diagonal crease on the ear lobe can be a risk factor for coronary artery disease and redness and tenderness of the pinna is a clue to a rare but treatable autoimmune inflammation of blood vessels in the brain. In rugby players and boxers complaining of memory loss I now always look specifically for cauliflower ears. Five years ago a young banker from the City complaining of a 'moving ear' was referred to me by a colleague working at the Royal National Ear Nose and Throat hospital on Gray's Inn Road. On examining him the only abnormality was that his left ear elevated and retracted involuntarily. He was emphatic that he had no control over the movement which continued as he spoke to me. I saw him several times after that and there was no improvement, so after informed consent I injected his auricularis superior and auricularis posterior muscles with a small amount of botulinum toxin. Within a few days his movements stopped and never returned. Late in my career the neurology of the human ear had become a fascinating new topic of interest.

In 2021, between coronavirus-imposed lockdowns, I set off with the vague intention of re-examining the emotional terrain of the Kings Road. People on the Tube were wearing face masks which highlighted the different shapes of their ears. After I had walked past invisible venues and dead avenues I was drawn to a chic boutique, brilliant white in the sunshine and contrasting sharply with the solid London brick of Radnor Mansions that rose from its roof. I went inside and was greeted by an elegant red-haired woman in a black silk dress wearing scarlet lipstick who followed me around the studio. After I had broken the ice by asking her if her dress was Jacquard, I took a chance and asked her, in French, if she had had her recent baby at home in Brittany. I could tell she had recently given birth because she still had some dark patches of chloasma on her temples and I noticed that her nails were bitten to the quick and there was a sadness in her eyes, raising the possibility of a recovering post-natal depression. Her red hair and freckles pointed to her being a Breton of Celtic descent. I then asked her if she knew who Zadig was, and she replied that he was the owner of the shop. Browsing the shelves between the travertine in Zadig & Voltaire created a timelessness that was marred only by the discreet black camera in the corner above the changing room. The other female assistant in the shop was much older and wore a silver cotton jacket. She had no wrinkles, but her face looked as if its normal contours had been smoothed away and there was a dry puffiness under her eyes. Up close, when I was paying at the desk, I noticed that her eyebrows were sparse and her cheeks slightly flushed. I was certain she had undiagnosed Myxoedema but I resisted a bystander diagnosis. As I left the shop she held her arms across her chest as if she was feeling the cold.

Not long after Sherlock Holmes meets Watson for the first time he tells him: 'A client is to me a mere unit, a factor in a problem', and Watson later describes his friend in *The Sign of the Four* as 'a calculating machine' and 'an automaton', detached from the world and without a social life. In 'The Adventure of the Mazarin Stone' Holmes pronounces: 'I am a brain, Watson.

The rest of me is a mere appendix.' Conan Doyle created a fictitious world in which all of its mysteries could be made to surrender their secrets to the intellect, and in which personal sorrow was appeased by a belief in eternal life. A neurologist who makes decisions shaped by wishful thinking is dealt with harshly by the General Medical Council, while trafficking in certitude and presenting data with triumphant finality, as Holmes was inclined to do, is now frowned upon. Medicine begins with the circumstances surrounding the case – colourful, lively and painful – and with it an acknowledgement that the lives of individuals who present with distressing and frightening symptoms are much more richly detailed than their symptoms suggest. No matter what Holmes uncovered through his careful appraisal of the evidence, his brooding on his store of case narratives, and his skill in reasoning backwards, much that was human was left out.

– Resurrection –

There were no hospital case notes nor general practitioner's records to go with the last brain that had been salvaged from the Maida Vale vaults. All I had to go on was a name, a date of birth and death, and a hospital in the northwest of England. When in 1995 I lifted it carefully out of its dusty white tub and cradled it in my gloved hands, it still had plenty of bounce. Its bloodless arteries did not feel hardened, and there were no patches of softening or signs of haemorrhage on its sand-coloured surface. It was no longer alive, but it was too magnificent to be dead. Its coralline ridges and intertidal folds resembled a marshy delta viewed from the sky. It was different from any other brain I had felt. This unknown tangible life was a symbolic legacy which epitomised the eighty years of good work that had been done at Maida Vale Hospital.

The brain had not lost weight, but it was impossible to tell that it was male and Caucasian. Under the attentive eye of Dr Susan Daniel I picked up my scalpel and separated the brainstem and the hind brain from the hemispheres. I next located the mamillary bodies and split the brain in two with a machete. The black stuff in the midbrain and the blue spot in the pons were missing. I also observed that the top of the brain-stem had shrunk, the globus pallidus was small and had orange-brown discolouration, the third and fourth ventricles and the aqueduct of Sylvius had expanded and there was thinning of the dentate nucleus in the cerebellar hemisphere. Dr Daniel then drew my attention to the fact that the subthalamic nucleus, a small almond-shaped structure in the basement of the brain, was less than half its usual size. Tissue was then extracted from several brain regions for further careful examination under the microscope. The technicians embedded each of these samples in paraffin wax, cut them into flat transparent slices with a fine steel blade and floated them out on the surface of warm water. The wafer-thin slivers were dried and then stained individually with haematoxylin and eosin, Bielschowsky silver impregnation and some with a new antiserum that marked an abnormal protein called tau. Once this was complete, each of the sections was mounted on a slide and protected with a glass coverslip.

Three weeks later I pulled out the three black rectangular boxes containing the slides and, using a bright field microscope with two eyepieces, began my examination by looking at the cellular detail of the anterior and posterior frontal cortex before plunging down into the basal ganglia to examine the nerve cells of the caudate and lenticular nuclei, the thalamus and the substantia nigra. Finally I turned my attention to the slides made from the lower brainstem and cerebellum. The zones that we had noted to be shrunken with the naked eye had lost large numbers of neurones and some of the surviving nerve cells contained spherical fibrillary tangles that reminded me of squash rackets. In other areas, the dying neurofilaments took the shape of flames. Pencil-like threads and comma shapes stained with silver were present in the subthalamic nucleus and the deep white matter. There was a profusion of star-shaped tufts, intermingled with radial fibrous arrays within astrocytes, and clumps of insoluble tau overloaded with phosphorus clogging up axons in the frontal cortex, the basal ganglia and the dentate ribbon. Our suspicions that had been based on naked eye examination of the brain were confirmed: Mr J.T. had lived his last years with a degenerative malady called Richardson's syndrome.

The monthly Grand Round held in the Wolfson Lecture Theatre of the National Hospital, Queen Square, continues to be a popular teaching session designed to teach aspirant neurologists the value of brain-cutting and the continuing usefulness of clinical-pathological correlation. The medical history of patients who had donated their brains for pathological examination are presented by research fellows familiar with the diagnosis. Sometimes when I was in the chair I would interrupt to make a teaching point or ask one of the junior doctors in the audience a question relating to the symptoms. I would then turn to one of the experts

on the front row to get their views on the case. When
the class had agreed on the most likely diagnosis based
on the history and examination the neuropatholo-
gists, Dr Tamas Revesz and Dr Susan Daniel, would
reveal the findings of the post-mortem examination,
always beginning with the macroscopic appearance
of the brain and spinal cord before moving on to the
microsocopic findings. When they had identified co-
morbidities a discussion involving the neurologists
would often ensue in an attempt to determine which
of the abnormal pathologies was most likely to have
been responsible for the clinical picture. A mismatch
between the consensual diagnosis made by the audience and the pathological findings was common. In
these sessions we were all trying to learn from our mistakes but at the same time reassure ourselves. Mr J.T.'s
was the only brain in the bank where there was no clinical information so he was unsuitable for presentation.

I closed my eyes and tried to create a joined-up
medical narrative that would bring Mr J.T. back from
the dead. I wanted to know from where he came, to
understand how he had come to be where he was and
how much or how little of his past he had carried with
him. I imagined that he had just stopped breathing
in the middle of the night and in the morning he had
been taken by two porters to the mortuary at Whiston Hospital where the autopsy had taken place. The
pathologist had failed to determine the cause of death
but had carefully removed the brain and spinal cord

for further examination and arranged for them to be transported by courier in the panier of a motorbike to Maida Vale Hospital.

In the last few months of his life, Mr J.T. had been reluctant to drink fluids and had choked on his food. He had lost his voice and could only communicate by nodding his head to signify yes or no or by making a growling noise. Even when he was awake his eyelids remained closed and he was unable to open them on request. His breathing was shallow and irregular, and from time to time he would take deep inspiratory sighs. An indwelling catheter had been inserted above his pubis to drain his bladder of urine and he required regular enemas to reduce the risk of faecal impaction and overflow incontinence. When his family visited him at the hospital his eyes would sometimes briefly open, but they appeared bolted to his orbit in a fixed unblinking stare. He was emaciated and rigid and could hardly move, a prisoner of his own body. It took two nurses to turn him over every hour to avoid pressure sores.

Two years earlier he had been living at home with the support of his family. His wife had reported to the general practitioner that sometimes when he tried to lever himself up using the arms of the chair he would shoot forward like a rocket and end up in a crumpled heap on the carpet. His neck was permanently extended, and saliva poured from his open mouth. If he tried to feed himself, much of the food spilled down the front of his shirt. He spent his day silent and motionless staring out over his small back garden. When his wife asked him a question he would try to answer but his response was markedly delayed and his speech drawling and gruff. His granddaughter noticed that he could not look up or down with his eyes. Sometimes he became angry or cried for no reason and on other occasions he would make an involuntary humming sound that continued for hours.

Four years before his death in 1985 he was still able to walk without assistance, but his lurching upright gait resembled that of a dancing bear. His neck would twist involuntarily to one side, causing him to bump into furniture. Sometimes there would be a crash in the bedroom and his wife would find him lying on his back on the floor. Everything about him had become very slow. Those who knew him said he had aged ten years overnight and one or two of his friends suspected he had taken to the bottle. This was as far back as I could travel. I had been able to invent a pathography from my knowledge of Mr J.T.'s diseased brain, but I was also intrigued about his life before he had become a patient. Outside my office were white buckets containing formalin-fixed brains waiting to be cut and prepared for histological examination. Sometimes in the early evening sitting alone at my desk after the laboratory staff had gone home I could hear the hum of their afterlife. I sensed cities chained by the rust of habit; I pictured lives submerged in symbolism, culture and myth and the skeletons of ancient trees concealed below grey membranes. I mapped vestigial flight paths and sea lanes that were crowded with desires, hopes and fears; I wanted to know what no longer was and that which had passed but was still alive. Richardson's syndrome was only the final chapter in what Mr J.T. had once been.

Altamirage, a term first coined by the neurologist and exponent of Zen, Dr Jim Austin, in his book *Chase, Chance, and Creativity: The Lucky Art of Novelty*, refers to a special personal quality by which good luck is prompted by an individual's distinctive actions. In my 2017 book *Mentored by a Madman: The William Burroughs Experiment*, I wrote how this form of serendipity had helped me to fly crookedly in my curiosity for cures. It would now come to my rescue again and help me make more human the horror of Mr J.T.'s final degeneration.

At the age of six I had started to go to watch the Saints (St Helens Rugby Football Club) on my tricycle and had stood in a pen behind the goalposts with other small boys cheering our thirteen red-hooped heroes. We used to sing: 'Oh we ain't got a barrel of money, but we've still got Langfield and Honey, there's Dougie and Llew running 'em through side by side' to a Patsy Cline song. When I left for medical school in London, this game I had watched growing up became a metaphor for the North of England, a piece of open-air theatre played under hard skies against a backdrop of factories, smoking chimneys and coal pits. It became a living symbol of the toughness and industry I associated with my birthplace; a remedy for homesickness and a protection from smug condescension.

Several years after I had divined Mr J.T.'s medical history, I was watching a Pathé newsreel on YouTube which featured the 1956 Rugby League Challenge Cup Final. The broadcaster had a very plummy voice and his banal colourless commentary made me laugh: 'Up for the cup. 80,000 Northern fans invaded Wembley for a real Roses battle, with St Helens, the Lancastrians, hoping to avert a fifth successive final defeat. Halifax, in the hooped jerseys, have the ball and attack. Wilkinson back-heels the ball to Palmer who passes to McIntyre but is brought to the ground by Rhodes.'

One of the St Helens players was called Mr J.T. In the first few minutes he opened Halifax's front door with a storming break, before being dragged to the floor by three men, one holding his legs, another who, as he fell to the ground, gave him a stiff arm to his windpipe and a third who went in with his shoulder. The game went back and forth with each team probing for their opponent's defensive weaknesses, using 'up and unders' and clever blind side breaks to get to the right end of the field. J.T. was raked and stamped on several times but he kept getting up. In the second half, the momentum seemed to be moving in the Saints' favour. J.T. took a pass, handed off the scrum half and bullocked down the middle before delivering an exquisite, measured pass to Llewellyn, the right centre, who sprinted thirty yards unopposed and laid the ball down beneath the posts.

J.T.'s surname was not uncommon on Merseyside, but I was able to learn from archival copies of the *St Helens Star* that the rugby league star had exactly the same date of birth as the rescued brain and that he had died in Whiston Hospital in 1991. I then read his obituary in the *Guardian* and ordered a copy of his death certificate from the General Register Office. The few available photographs online showed a tough-looking, brawny man with a thin face, brown tousled hair, cauliflower ears, a long angular jaw and a missing front tooth. The obituary said that he had been born in St Helens and his Irish father had worked at Pilkington's glassworks. At school he had built up his strength by scrummaging against a brick wall that bordered the playing fields and before he became a professional footballer he had worked as a collier. When he finished his shift he would run several miles, twice a week, to train with the team. On one occasion, when playing for Great Britain against the Kangaroos in Sydney, he broke his wrist but refused to leave the pitch. For those who had watched him play he was ferocious and brave, but those who knew him vouched for his gentleness and sense of humour. After finishing his playing career at Warrington he had returned to St Helens to coach 'the little angels' at Blackbrook. I also learned from biographical sketches that during his time as a miner he had gone to art classes and had continued to paint and draw local scenes throughout his life. His musical tastes included brass band fantasias and Tchaikovsky and he raced homing pigeons. On his death certificate cerebral degeneration was given as the likely cause of his demise

By using my imagination and suspending my belief in the gospel of science I had created a fresh focus. I had established a continuum between J.T.'s brain-hood and the astrocytic tufts I had looked at under the microscope, but all the same I regretted that I had never been able to talk with him, especially before he became unwell. I also began to worry how long the seeds of Richardson's syndrome had been lying dormant in his brain before they had started to engulf him.

– Machine Learning –

When brain scanning arrived in the late nineteen-seventies, I welcomed it as another way of validating my clinical method. I returned to the light boxes, where I had learned to read skull X-rays and sat in on meetings conducted in dark rooms in the basement of Queen Square. Nuclear magnetic resonance imaging depended on the fact that humans are composed of water and fat and that each of the body's hydrogen atoms behaves like a gyroscope in a magnetic field. Radiofrequency pulses with a specific frequency are able to flip hydrogen protons, and as they relax back to their original position photons of energy are released that induce detectable signals. This data is then fed into a computer to make a grid of millions of pixels which are represented in the image on the screen by three-dimensional blocks called voxels. One of the neuroradiologists brought two spinning tops in to help me understand the rudiments of quantum mechanics.

As I looked at these brand-new reproductions, I started to appreciate the diseased nervous system in a completely different light. I was now able to visualise plaques of demyelination in the living brain, measure the size of the hippocampus in suspected Alzheimer's disease and know within less than an hour whether a stroke had resulted from a blood clot or a brain haemorrhage. In contrast to computerised axial tomography (CT scans), a slightly earlier and equally miraculous innovation, no radiation was involved. These two new scanners eradicated the need for painful and invasive procedures like myelography and air encephalograms.

My colleagues in the department of neuroradiology were now helping me to acquire a new imagination and a different gaze. I was observing pathology through a set of abnormal physical signals and approximations. At each session they pointed out brain and spinal cord anomalies and aberrations that I had failed to notice, many of which had a direct bearing on the patient's symptoms. It felt like a momentous new beginning that would transform the practice of neurology. Ten years after I had started out as a neurologist, I needed to configure the dimensions of the brain in new sagittal, axial and coronal planes and learn new technical terminology and a list of sequences. Fortunately there was a bestiary of pareidolias that helped me to recognise and remember some of the abnormal radiological signs including, the eye of the tiger, the hummingbird, the giant panda, the leopard skin, the butterfly, the cod fish, the medusa, the swallowtail and the elephant. I was starting my clinical investigations all over again, learning to see a complementing picture.

Magnetic resonance imaging, although expensive,

soon became routine. The new 1.5 Tesla machines had a flux density thirty thousand times greater than the earth's magnetic field, created by an electrical charge circulating through a superconductor and cooled by liquid helium. Brain surgeons joked that an MR scanner was more valuable than fifty neurologists. But during those reporting sessions I had attended in the early days my neuroradiological colleagues had told me that in the absence of a request form that provided precise details of the tempo and nature of the patient's symptoms they would be unable to advise the radiographers and technicians on the correct MR sequences and that later when looking at the images distinguish the wood from the trees. The findings on imaging, as in the neurological examination, were never clear cut.

The majority of patients I see in clinic have symptoms beyond the resolution of even the most powerful brain scanner. At the end of each consultation, when the time comes to decide if tests are needed, I run the following questions through my head: 'What am I looking for with the test?' 'If it is present, how will it influence my final diagnosis and management?' And, most importantly, 'Will the finding ultimately benefit the patient?' The threshold I set is sufficiently high that the chance of incidental findings is outweighed by the likelihood of finding a diagnostically useful abnormality. If I feel a scan is needed in an elderly person where the frequency of abnormal signals is much higher, I explain that the brain, in common with skin, acquires blemishes during life and may also possess longstanding birthmarks and cysts that have no bearing on the current symptoms and require no intervention. Over time I have learned to ask better questions of the scans I order and at the same time reduce the number of anxious victims of modern imaging technology. If a patient is dissatisfied with my clinical diagnosis and insists on a brain scan I usually accede to the request once I have gone over with them the downsides to the procedure.

The following story illustrates how a 'flipped physical' when imaging is ordered prior to seeing a patient is not only profligate and bad practice but can even lead to error. Mr U., a man in his late seventies, came to see me for his regular annual follow-up at Queen Square, where I had been treating him for tremor for fifteen years. He was keen to tell me about some headaches that had started in Florida during the summer. He described a feeling of having a tight band around the top of his head that built up over an hour or so and which tended to be worse in the early evening. He had not noticed any triggers for the discomfort, but commented that two paracetamol tablets helped relieve it. He also mentioned that his hands had been shaking a lot more since the headaches started. A few weeks before his scheduled return to England he had been in so much pain that he had contacted the local hospital in Boca Raton and had been put through to a neurologist. Over the phone he was told that he needed to have an urgent magnetic resonance brain scan to exclude a tumour or a brain haemorrhage. On arrival at the hospital he was asked to fill in copious forms and provide his credit card details, before being directed to the imaging suite.

Encased inside the MR machine he found the loud banging, whirring and clanging noises due to the vibrating metal coils extremely distressing, but managed to keep his head still and refrain from pressing the escape button. The scan took about an hour and he then went for blood tests. A nurse asked him to fill out some more tick-box forms relating to his general health, past medical and family history, as well as two detailed headache questionnaires. After waiting outside the neurologist's office for a few minutes he was buzzed in. The neurologist was sitting in a high revolving chair behind a huge desk on which there was a computer and a mobile phone. A number of framed diplomas and certificates hung on the wall. After the most cursory and businesslike greeting, Mr U. was told that he had three 'UBOs' (unidentified bright objects) on his scan and that further tests were needed to investigate whether they were caused by cerebrovascular disease, head trauma or multiple sclerosis. Pleased that something had shown up he had no hesitation in agreeing to an ultrasound of his carotid arteries, magnetic resonance angiography and a full cardiological work up that included electrocardiograms, an echocardiogram, more blood tests and an opinion from a heart specialist. The full assessment was completed in seventy-two hours. On returning to see the neurologist he was relieved to be told that the tests had come back normal, but that he would need to have repeat scans and blood tests in six months' time and that he may also need a spinal tap.

Mr U. described what had happened to him in great detail and was effusive about the speed and thoroughness of the investigations. He was also relieved that a brain tumour had been excluded, but after two weeks his headaches had returned and he was now also anxious to talk to me about the cause of the bright objects on the scan. His wife then pulled out a several pages long computerised medical report. On the first page there were four lines devoted to the medical history, followed by a very long list of uninformative negative test findings. The next page listed the results of all the investigations he had received and was riddled with unintelligible acronyms. The long-winded magnetic resonance imaging report described in minute detail three small areas of hyperintensity in the basement of the brain and a large number of normal findings but came to no conclusion. After wading through another page of padding I turned to the last paragraphs hoping to understand what the neurologist had thought about Mr U.'s presenting symptoms. 'Scan negative headache' was given as the diagnosis with a recommendation that further tests would be needed. There was no mention at all about his long-standing tremor.

Mr U. told me that the neurologist in Florida had not examined him and so I asked him to lie down on the couch. I began by feeling his head and palpating his temporal arteries before pressing on his sinuses, checking his jaw movements and looking at the back of his eyes. I then examined his ear drums with my otoscope, and deliberately listened over his carotid arteries and eyes for bruits, even though I knew his blood vessels had been imaged. I took his pulse, checked for heart murmurs and measured his blood pressure both lying down and after standing up for two minutes. After he had sat down and I had recorded my findings I told him that the bright dots on the scan were red herrings. I went on to say that there was little doubt that he was experiencing tension headaches and that I recommended he cut back a little on coffee, take regular exercise and investigate techniques to relax his mind. A month later he returned to the clinic and told me that the headaches had gone and his long-standing tremor had settled down. In the course of our conversation he also told me that he had finally managed to sell the family business to a decent individual who he had every confidence would run it properly.

I kept my views on his management in Boca Raton to myself but felt that even if the neurologist had considered a scan to be essential, he should have told Mr U. that there was a significant chance of the brain scan throwing up incidental findings and that he should also have refrained from mentioning the possibility of a brain tumour over the phone. A normal scan may serve as a temporary placebo, but the reporting of incidental anomalies can cause unnecessary worry that does not disappear, even after reassurances that the imaging findings are of no clinical significance. Eight out of ten patients with episodic headaches in neurological practice do not require a brain scan and I would not have ordered one in Mr U.'s case. On the other hand, in about one in every ten scans that I order I get a salutary reminder of the fallibility of my clinical methods when something totally unexpected shows up and changes my diagnosis.

Private hospitals are there to generate income and all the rhetoric of quality, safety and patient satisfaction is in truth no more than a public relations exercise. In common with psychoanalysis, a medical setting and on-site medical expertise are not necessary to perform magnetic resonance imaging. This has resulted in a loosening of the ties between the medical indications for carrying out a scan and the motives for performing it. It is natural for a commercial company or a health-care organisation to want their expensive equipment to pay its way and, hopefully, turn in a profit, but unfortunately financial gain often moves into conflict with clinical need, and the limitation of medically selected referrals becomes an obstacle. The neurological consultation is time-consuming and a low value has been attached to it. Most neurologists working in the private sector have been forced to become factory workers in what has become a service industry. Their efforts to be kind and treat the patient as an individual are stymied at every stage by an enterprise culture that follows the money.

Expensive technologies that need powerful magnets, cyclotron particle accelerators and proton beams are looked upon as a visible sign of prestige and excellence by university teaching hospitals. Most of the deans and directors of neurological institutes and heads of department are now divorced almost entirely from clinical practice. They are obliged to spend most of their time in administration signing forms and sitting on committees. They are under pressure to bring in new signings whose work is underpinned by large grants and to raise money for new buildings. Recently I was saddened to overhear one of these leaders of my profession say to a neuroscientist: 'All I need to know is whether my patient can walk or not, so that I can tick the box on the brain scan request form that asks me whether she is ambulant or requires a chair or stretcher.'

While medical technology has greatly enhanced the ability to diagnose and treat disease it has also encouraged a mental laziness in some doctors. These individuals, who are instantly recognisable to colleagues, have acquired, in the course of their training, a laboratory-orientated mindset. They are extremely proficient at ordering tests and procedures, but don't always know when they should be ordering them or how to interpret the results. Yoked to their machines they treat numbers rather than patients and revel in the measurement game. As a result of blunderbuss screening they conjure up brilliant diagnoses from time to time, but also leave in their wake a large number of casualties. Bryan Matthews, a clinician who became the Professor of Neurology in Oxford, anticipated this when he wrote in his book *Practical Neurology* in 1963: 'If investigations can be carried out by the signing of a form requesting someone else to do them, there is a temptation to obtain as much information as possible by this simple method.' These doctors with inattentional blindness never have time to listen or analyse their findings in relation to a patient's needs. The more insightful of them have the sense to move into a diagnostic speciality where they are rarely or never in contact with patients.

Although I believe that brain scans have had the largest positive impact on neurological practice in the last fifty years, there are other technological platforms that have added useful new dimensions to the diagnostic process. Electroencephalography provides tracings of brain waves that help neurologists decide whether a funny turn is due to epilepsy and where in the brain the abnormal focus of electrical activity is coming from. Nerve conduction studies and electromyography provide data on the speed of impulses along nerves and whether loss of nerve or muscle fibres has occurred. When these findings are combined with my clinical examination I can determine with far greater certainty whether weakness is due to muscle disease or a disorder affecting part of the peripheral nervous system. Clinical neurophysiology is one way to understand what goes wrong in the diseased nervous system, and in my early years I carried out this test myself, but then as pressure to see more patients increased and I became more specialised, I was reluctantly obliged to give it up and hand the privilege of turning on the power, activating 'the electronic stethoscope' and listening to the music over to a colleague. Blood and urine examinations allow me to diagnose rare inborn errors of metabolism and there are now laboratories to precisely characterise autonomic nervous system dysfunction, hearing and balance disorders and neurological causes of visual impairment. Medical genetics has changed the way I practise nosography as radically as Charcot did one hundred and fifty years ago. This new knowledge lies beyond the resolution of the electron microscope at the molecular level and has started to affect the way I think about the cause of disease. The identification of abnormal genes and molecules has led to the development of new therapies like ribonucleic acid (RNA) interference and antisense oligonucleotides that can modify the course of hitherto untreatable disorders like muscular dystrophy, familial amyloid neuropathy and spinal muscular atrophy.

My clinical gaze has been forced to embrace new

anatomical, metabolic, electrical and chemical vistas. The images these create in my mind are as strange and wonderful as maps of the dark side of the moon. Many are exquisitely beautiful, but more importantly they provide insight into the nature of brain disease beyond anything I could have imagined at the start of my training. I now visualise the brain as a tapestry in different spatial dimensions. I see swirling coronas, moving dots, starbursts of crimson alpha rhythms and axonal twinkling highways that resemble São Paulo from the air at night.

The evidence-based portals on the world wide web have now replaced the long hours I used to spend going through filing cabinets, chasing references in *Index Medicus* and looking up facts in textbooks in the hope of tracking down the cause of a patient's unexplained and undiagnosed symptoms. Although my mobile phone is switched off while I am listening to the patient's medical history, applications that record tremor frequency and scales to measure the degree of cognitive impairment have become useful additions to my digital toolbox. I can also now review a patient's video clips, and with permission record their physical signs on the phone.

The internet has also changed the medical consultation in an extraordinary way. An eighteen-year-old university student came to see me complaining of progressive loss of hearing, a ringing sound in the ears, severe headaches and blurred vision. Her mother, who had come with her to the consultation, added that her daughter's behaviour had changed in the last few months. She was now unable to concentrate on her studies and had developed a persecution complex. After taking a full history and carrying out a detailed examination I was about to explain that, on examining the back of the eye, I had noticed there was a blockage in one of the branches of her retinal artery, when her mother piped up: 'Professor Lees, we have googled Francesca's symptoms and wonder if she might have SUSAC syndrome?' She then told me that it was an autoimmune condition that affects very small blood vessels in the brain, inner ear and retina and which can be treated with intravenous immunoglobulin and corticosteroids. She next handed me some printed copies of the pertinent medical literature to read later.

Over the years, family members and nurses had given me vital information that gifted me a patient's diagnosis, and patients have provided clues as to what might be the most appropriate treatment, but this was a totally new twenty-first-century variant on William Osler's maxim: 'Listen to your patient, she is telling you the diagnosis.' I had not just been beaten to the punch, but had been introduced, for the first time, to a disease I had never encountered.

Confronted with a constellation of mysterious clinical symptoms that I do not recognise, I also use Google. Sometimes when I type the key words in, a disorder with an instantly forgettable name such as

'PLA2G6-associated neurodegeneration' pops up and genetic testing then proves it to be correct. I have also learned how to scroll through digital brain scan images and actively access laboratory investigations on my computer.

The great age of diagnosis where reputations were made by identifying 'black swans' at the bedside has passed, and neurology's focus has rightly shifted to the better treatment of chronic disease. Looking and listening are no longer the vaunted skills they once were when the armamentarium to treat neurological disorders was threadbare. Ironically, as health technology with its veneer of certainty has advanced and more therapies have become available, patients have become ever more desperate to be heard and for their laments to be both listened to by someone they trust, and then acted upon in private. I have found that the more machinery I have at my disposal the greater the demands have become on my clinical judgement. The most thorough clinical examination is required for the many patients where my medical history suggests that there is no organic neurological disorder, or where no structural damage has been found on imaging.

Technology remains the servant of clinical reason and not its fulcrum. I continue to resist a strictly engineering approach to neurology and consider defensive medicine, including the profligate use of brain scanning, a form of medical malpractice. From time to time

I also remind myself of what Richard Asher warned me about when I was studying for my postgraduate exams: 'Even if you own a computer it is advisable to spend a certain amount of time in thought.' Although the internet is a great leveller it has also become the most potent anxiety-provoking system mankind has yet to devise.

Every day at the hospital I learn something new that transcends facts and makes me question my decisions. By chatting to my patients I learn about their gestalt as well as the colour of their feathers. The less time I spend trying to decipher the latest medical science, the better listener – and better neurologist – I become. A hypochondriasis that first emerged during my training ensures that I continue to treat people with the tenderness I would expect from my own doctors. I also continue to go beyond clinical guidelines if I believe my actions are in the interest of the patient. Through endless non-linear discovery of nature's secrets and the continued observation of birds and plants, I have become better able to deal with the arbitrary and often brutal nature of neurological illness.

– Acknowledgements –

ll patients' names have been changed to preserve anonymity. Mr J.T. did not exist, although a brain with no clinical details found to have Richardson's syndrome did. The method of working backwards from death to life I describe is an attempt to try to imagine brainhood.

My patients are the first to thank because even in the autumn of my career they continue to be my most important source of inspiration. Gerald Stern was the piston for my lasting love affair with neurology. Hardly a week goes by without me thinking of something he taught me. The extramural passions of Proust, cosmology, Stephenson's Rocket, calligraphy, brain failure in public life and Mauritius – which William Gooddy brought to the Wednesday ward rounds – were influential in my desire to write imaginatively and in my evolving naturalistic and holistic credo. As an outsider excluded from the inner crucible of British neurology, Gooddy also quietly encouraged me to challenge hierarchies and pull up some of the props that sustained them.

I am grateful to the physicians who took a special interest in me and showed me how to be a neurologist. In chronological order they are Ronald Henson, Christopher Earl, John Marshall, Michael Harrison, Peter Gautier Smith and MacDonald Critchley. All of these men are dead, but what they taught me lives on forever. I also wish to thank colleagues and friends who have helped me with my historical lacunes, given their own opinions and put the record straight where my imagination had got the better of me. My gratitude in alphabetical order goes to Yves Agid, Alastair Compston, Denis Donovan, Bruno Dubois, Rolf Jager, Hadi Manji, Timothy Nicholson, Werner Poewe, Jacques Poirier, Nikolas Rose, Tamas Revesz, Jon Stone, Michael Swash, Olivier Walusinski and Michael Zandi. Some of the themes in this book have been partly covered in learned journals, and I wish to acknowledge the editorial encouragement of Tehseen Noorani at the *Polyphony*, Masud Husain at *Brain* and Elena Becker-Barroso at the *Lancet*.

Three extraordinary institutions have played an important part in my career. Firstly The London Hospital, Whitechapel, which provided me with a solid medical training; then University College Hospital that gave me a second chance after I had abandoned hope of ever becoming a neurologist; and finally to my surprise the National Hospital, Queen Square, whose board appointed me as a consultant at the age of thirty-three, providing me with further opportunity to learn through interaction with its staff of brilliant clinicians. Feedback from my many research fellows taught me that a story replete with human interest was much more educational than an intangible fact.

I also want to thank my wife Juana for her forbearance during the many evenings I have spent in the company of my mistress, Lady Neurology, and for ensuring my feet never leave the ground.

Editors are so important that I think their contribution should be acknowledged on a book's front cover. Rosalind Porter at Notting Hill Editions reminded me of the importance of chronology, tempo and clarity as I made my final revisions; her thoughtful and knowledgeable edits will also allow this book to be read through without the need for a medical dictionary and a textbook of neurology. My thanks also to Anthony Mercer for exceptional copy-editing. I also wish to thank Kim Kremer for publishing what can be seen as a follow-up to *Mentored by a Madman: The William Burroughs Experiment*.

Thanks go to Sara Lawson at the Queen Square Library Archives for providing the photograph of Maida Vale Hospital, to Barts Health Archives and Museums for the picture of Clifford Wilson teaching a group of medical students at The London Hospital, and to Dr Olivier Walusinksi for permission to reproduce a copy of the Brouillet tableau depicting Charcot and his assistants and the patient Blanche Wittman.

The Caffè Tropea, Bar Italia, The Lady Ottoline and The Manette Cafe in London's West End are four important locations where I have observed the panoply of abnormal human behaviour during some of my writing.